Early Praise for *What It's L*

" A must read! Dr. Moeller's fascinating dissection of the intricacies involved in becoming a physician and the hurdles that a young doctor must overcome gets an A+ in Gross Anatomy 101 of the healthcare system. His unique insight, wit, and intelligent analysis of the multi-billion dollar debacle we call healthcare does not cease to draw the reader in. Ultimately, Dr. Moeller provides a view that only a well-versed medical doctor can provide and allows us to understand the trials and tribulations of the select few who truly devote their life to their passion: healing humankind."

AMIT BHAN, MD, Henry Ford Health System, Detroit, MI

"This book by Dr. Moeller describes the real journey of becoming a doctor. Dr. Moeller's experiences are representative of the real day-to-day challenges physicians face. The enormous sacrifice required to become a physician and the burden of managing all of the complexities of practicing medicine has not been presented to the public the way Dr. Moeller describes it in his book. I think this book is a great read, true to the core, and is sure to provide a unique perspective on what it takes to be a doctor for anyone who is not already in this profession."

EUGENE ZOLOTAREVSKY, MD, Ypsilanti, MI

"This book is a gripping profile of the sacrifices, both personal and financial, it takes to become a highly specialized physician. The general public and lawmakers in Congress, in particular, could greatly benefit from reading this book. Dr. Moeller also dispels several myths regarding physicians—most importantly the one that professes that all physicians are rich. He also provides a detailed analysis on how to 'fix' the healthcare system so physicians can focus more time on taking care of patients and less time on meaningless paperwork and the other daily frustrations that have nothing to do with patient care. These issues are leading so many physicians to leave medicine or retire early."

GREGORY OLDS, MD, Chattanooga, TN

"Dr. Moeller takes the reader on an insider's journey of what it takes to be a physician in this day and age. Through his keen insight, one can appreciate the rigorous academic schedule and the tireless hours of the internship, residency, and fellowship. It includes humanistic accounts of personal sacrifices and the emotional rollercoaster that is interwoven into the life of a contemporary physician. The book culminates with an intelligent explanation of the economics of healthcare. He exquisitely explains that what a physician actually gets paid is quite different from the charges patients see on their bill and reminds us that the tireless attention to patients' well-being via phone calls (even at 3 a.m.) and family consultations are not accounted for in a doctor's compensation—there isn't overtime pay in medicine.

"Without regret, Dr. Moeller, like many of his colleagues, commits to the profession of medicine because of the altruistic nature inherent to the role and the intellectual stimulation afforded by the practice. Overall, this book provides a sobering perspective of healthcare providers on the front lines of medicine, and a call to action that would include the voices of these front line providers in the ongoing reform of the U.S. healthcare system."

NICK LIBERATI, Reimbursement Specialist, Grand Rapids, MI

"Medicine is considered a noble profession because of what we, as physicians, have to sacrifice for our patients and society. This book has done a wonderful job of portraying the rigors of what it takes to become a physician and offers potential solutions that reference the principles of our founding fathers and free market economics, the pillars of what makes the United States so great. It is both an emotional portrait of the life of physicians as well as truly patriotic!"

PRASHANT KRISHNAN, MD, Colorado Springs, CO

"The life of a physician is not an easy one. This book highlights the enormous struggle, sacrifice, and commitment necessary to become a physician and the real-life challenges physicians face when they are in practice. As a nurse, I recognize there are many current issues in healthcare that need to be addressed. It is my sincere hope that this is read by not only members of the general public so that there may be a better understanding and appreciation of physicians, but also by legislators who can affect the policy changes that need to occur. "

LISA GABIER, Staff Nurse, Grand Rapids, MI

"Dr. Moeller's book is a fun read and an accurate depiction of the training involved in the evolution of an American physician. Dr. Moeller draws insight to many of the flaws in our current healthcare system and offers some creative solutions. This book is a must-read for politicians and hospital administrators."

DANIALD RODRIGUES, MD, Fellowship, Wayne State University

"As a patient of Dr. Matthew Moeller, I can now see the challenges of becoming a physician and the continued challenges physicians face in their career. It is astounding how much work is placed on them to complete this journey into helping others attempt to live a better life. The handicaps placed on them and the burdens they face throughout the course of their lives and their family's lives to help society as a whole is proof of the compelling need for some policy makers to actually involve them in the decision-making process."

MICHEAL CORREALE, Patient, Lansing, MI

"Dr. Moeller's book is a must-read for everyone who is interested in attending medical school. The insight he provides into the journey of the medical profession is unparalleled. Dr. Moeller deserves tremendous accolades for taking the time and articulating his opinions on the current problems in healthcare. More Dr. Moellers are necessary for a successful, efficient, and affordable American healthcare system for the 21st century."

RANDALL MEISNER, MD, Fellowship, University of Wisconsin

"It seems as if public's perception of doctors has been relatively negative in recent years and perhaps motivated by the media and the current state of politics in the nation. Dr. Moeller accurately portrays 'our side' and rekindles the notions of service, dedication, and nobility to the medical profession that seem not to be noticed amongst politicians lately."

PRAVEEN SATEESH, MD, Fellowship, Georgetown University

What It's Like to Become a Doctor

THE YEAR-BY-YEAR JOURNEY FROM MEDICAL STUDENT TO PRACTICING PHYSICIAN

MATTHEW MOELLER, MD

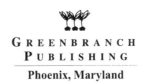

GREENBRANCH
PUBLISHING

Phoenix, Maryland

PO Box 208
Phoenix, MD 21131
Phone: (800) 933-3711
Fax: (410) 329-1510
Email: info@greenbranch.com
Websites: www.greenbranch.com, www.mpmnetwork.com, www.soundpractice.net,
www.codapedia.com

No patent liability is assumed with respect to the use of the information contained herein. Although every precaution has been taken in the preparation of this book, the publisher and the authors assume no responsibility for errors or omissions. Nor is any liability assumed from damages resulting from the use of the information contained herein. For information, Greenbranch Publishing, PO Box 208, Phoenix, MD 21131.

This book includes representations of the author's personal experiences and do not reflect actual patients or medical situations.

This book is not intended as a substitute for the medical advice of physicians. The reader should regularly consult a physician in matters relating to his/her health and particularly with respect to any symptoms that may require diagnosis or medical attention.

The strategies contained herein may not be suitable for every situation. This publication is designed to provide general medical practice management information and is sold with the understanding that neither the author nor the publisher is engaged in rendering legal, accounting, ethical, or clinical advice. If legal or other expert advice is required, the services of a competent professional person should be sought.

CPT™® is a registered trademark of the American Medical Association.

Greenbranch Publishing books are available at special quantity discounts for bulk purchases as premiums, fund-raising, or educational use. info@greenbranch.com or (800) 933-3711.

13   8 7 6 5 4 3 2 1

Copyedited, typeset, and printed in the United States of America

PUBLISHER
Nancy Collins

EDITORIAL ASSISTANT
Jennifer Weiss

BOOK DESIGNER
Laura Carter
Carter Publishing Studio

COPYEDITOR
Pat George

Table of Contents

About the Author

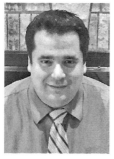 Matthew Moeller, MD, is a double board-certified physician in Internal Medicine and Gastroenterology. He is the author of several peer-reviewed scientific articles in *Gastroenterology* and *Hepatology* and has spoken on topics of liver and gastroenterology diseases in national and international forums. He is a member of the prestigious Alpha Omega Alpha Honor Society awarded to the top medical students in terms of academic success and community service, and a member of Phi Beta Kappa, a selective honor society awarded to top college students in terms of aptitude. Trained at the University of Michigan and at Henry Ford in Detroit., he currently practices Gastroenterology in Michigan. He enjoys spending time with his wife and four children, including participating in school and sporting activities.

Acknowledgements

First, I dedicate this book to my current and future patients. I put my heart and soul into my patients daily and I hope that my book can translate into positive changes to our healthcare system. Second, I thank my wife, Jackie, who has been patient and supportive, yet given me the fuel to continue to pursue my dreams as a physician and author. Third, I thank my parents, who have given me the tools that I need to succeed. Finally, I thank my colleagues, including nurses, doctors, and medical staff, who are the engines that make quality patient care possible.

Introduction

I AM A 34-YEAR-OLD GASTROENTEROLOGIST, ONE YEAR OUT OF fellow-ship. I am employed in a large medical system in Michigan. With this detailed account of my journey from student to board-certified gastro-enterologist, I hope to accomplish three goals:

1. Enlighten young minds and aspiring doctors about the challenging yet rewarding path to becoming a doctor. I walk the reader through this journey, step by step, year by year, beginning with my senior year of high school, opening a window to the daily life of a medical student, intern, resident, and fellow. My wish is that this book will enlighten America's future doctors, but also make them aware of the obstacles and sacrifices they will encounter in this rewarding career should they choose this path.

2. Educate lawmakers about the sacrifices and hardships doctors face so they can better understand why decisions about healthcare should be made by, or at least with the input of, practicing doctors rather than politicians. Unless lawmakers are familiar with the financial, intellectual, social, mental, and physical challenges of the profession, how can they truly know what reforms are necessary?

   A strength of this book is that it presents the perspective of a doctor on the front lines of medicine, a regular practicing doctor who has tasted his own sweat and tears during his journey. It was not written by a Congressman who used to be a doctor, or a doctor who now lobbies in Washington, D.C., or a hospital administrator who has never treated a sick patient.

3. Educate the public about a doctor's reality so they can better understand the challenges we face as we strive to provide them with the quality of care they deserve. My goal is to show patients that we dedicate our hearts, minds, and souls to our work every day, making sacrifices of our own so we can make their lives healthier.

In addition, I hope to clarify some misconceptions about doctors from a social and financial standpoint, including misconceptions about patient bills, doctors' reimbursement methods, and unique tax laws. I hope that my insight changes the perceptions of doctors as rich, omnipotent, and emotionless, illustrating, instead, that they are regular people who work hard, have families, and experience the same emotions, challenges, and weaknesses as everyone else.

I also offer solutions to our current healthcare crisis that would benefit patients, doctors, and society.

CHAPTER 1

Call Night, December 2012

I T'S 3:00 A.M. AND THE COLORFUL MONITORS in my patient's ICU room are beeping in no recognizable pattern. A familiar rerun of "M.A.S.H." is playing at low volume on the small TV above the patient's bed, which is basically a convention for late-night calls to patients' rooms. Fresh blood speckles the ceiling and the recognizable odors of stool and blood envelop the room.

I sit down on a chair and feel my scrub shirt soaked with sweat as I remove my gown. I then waddle like a duck over to a computer along the wall, careful not to slip in the fresh blood that is pooling on the floor. My efforts to log in the procedure I just performed are in vain—the system is down. I look over at my patient, who is lying on his back, sedated, with blood dripping off the corners of his mouth. I do a quick check. His chest is rising. The monitors show all his vital signs are stable. The nurses are cleaning up the blood around his mouth and recording vital signs.

The system is still down. I find a pen and document what I just did on a piece of paper in the patient's chart: "s/p EGD, large bleeding esophageal varices, s/p 6 bands placed. Start IV ABX, continue octreotide gtt for 5 days, then start beta blocker." I look up the patient's phone number in the chart and call the family. Unfortunately, the number is disconnected. I try the alternate number. No answer. I ask the nurse what doctor is covering tonight. She is not certain, but gives me an extension. I call. No answer. I'll call him back in a few minutes.

I thank my nurses for their care and walk down the long yellow halls, peppered with the sounds of monitors going off in other patients' rooms. I wait for two sets of elevators, and then leave the hospital, walking through the cold, dark parking lot to my car. It's snowing hard—I slowly make my 20-minute drive home, hoping I get there before I get another call that will require me to turn around. My phone doesn't ring. I arrive home safely and crawl into bed. My adrenaline is still pumping. I had just saved a man's life.

Four hours earlier, I had been at home with my family, reading *'Twas the Night Before Christmas* to my four-year-old son, who was excited about Santa's impending visit. My other kids were watching "Elf" on TV. My wife was finishing up the dishes. Then, I got the page from a frantic resident physician (trainee) insisting I come to the hospital immediately. A patient with advanced liver disease had uncontrollable internal bleeding. He might need an urgent esophagogastroduodenoscopy. I kissed my wife and kids and headed out the door. Christmas Eve or not, I had a job to do.

And now, at home, in my bed, I try to get some much-needed sleep. However, instead of sugarplums dancing in my head, my mind conjures up visions of a large bleeding vessel spurting blood and a retching patient gasping for air. How did I get to this place?

CHAPTER 2

My Youth—The 1990s

I GREW UP IN A MIDDLE-CLASS FAMILY in Lake Orion, Michigan, a town of 3,000 people about 35 miles north of Detroit. My father was an information technology manager at General Motors and my mother was a school secretary in Lake Orion. I have three younger siblings: twin sisters and a brother.

When I was in elementary school, I longed to be an NBA basketball player. I lost that innocent eight-year-old fantasy when I realized I wasn't tall enough, and turned my sights on being a marine biologist. I read a lot about fish and marine life and even convinced my parents to buy me a 10-gallon aquarium. One day, noting that a fish in my tank was swimming awkwardly, I quickly retrieved him from my aquarium and attempted to use a basketball inflation needle to resuscitate him by blowing into the needle. I carefully placed him back into the aquarium and he swam away! I was convinced I had just saved that fish. I still remember that feeling of elation.

In fifth and sixth grade, I enjoyed doing science homework and loved reading about various species of fish. My parents thought it was interesting that I wanted to study the ocean, as I had never even seen the ocean. But my interests changed again in middle school. For my science project in seventh grade, I wanted to show how a heart beats and what happens when the arteries get clogged. My father, a talented handyman, took me to the hardware store to buy toilet tubing and a fishbowl. He explained that I could use the tubes as arteries and the fish bowl as the heart. Before we knew it, we had red colored water with a pump pushing water through the fish bowl. We inserted valves to cut off part of the flow to show what happens with heart disease. I called the project, "Simulation of the Circulating Heart."

After getting several awards for this project, I decided I wanted to be a doctor. "Doogie Howser, MD" was on primetime television then, and watching Doogie (Neil Patrick Harris) help others and seeing the satisfaction he felt inspired me. Plus, I thought he was pretty cool.

I enrolled at Brother Rice, an all-male Catholic high school known for its superior athletics and challenging academic curriculum. My parents and I thought this was a good fit—it would be challenging and would bring out the best in me. At Brother Rice, I took several science courses that reinforced my interest in and enthusiasm about the field of medicine. My parents said I simply enjoyed studying in general and had intrinsic motivation. While my friends played pick-up football games, I spent three to four hours in my room studying. There were about 10–15 students in my honors high school curriculum who were very competitive. That culture of competition ignited a fire inside of me that burned with passion to be better than the next guy. I wanted to be on top.

I remember dissecting a cat in my anatomy class my senior year of high school. My lab partner was surprised by how focused I was about learning all the cat's body parts. I saved the latissimus dorsi muscle and brought it home in my book bag. My parents thought that was strange, so it ended up in the trash.

As much as I studied, I still enjoyed a world beyond books. I was on the football team at Brother Rice. My outstanding coach, Al Fracassa, still inspires me to this day. He taught me more about life than about football. He instilled in me the desire to be the best that I can be. Coach Fracassa often exclaimed, "Do it better than it has ever been done!" I still hold this "never give up" attitude dear to my heart.

Our motto my junior year of high school was "Attitude Is Everything." Having the right attitude no matter what life throws at you can help you accomplish anything. During my junior year, I injured my knee while playing football and could not play for the rest of the year. I wanted to remain part of the team, so I continued to show up to practices. Despite my lack of any role on the field, Coach Fracassa still valued me and made me feel a part of the team. He said I had a great attitude toward life despite my setback. I used his teachings as a model for how to treat others in life: Be kind to everyone and find value in every person, no matter their role or position in life.

My interest in medicine continued in high school. I shadowed an Emergency Room doctor in a local hospital for several weeks, and after watching him perform some interesting procedures and treat sick people, combined with my academic success in high school, I decided that medicine really was my calling.

Early in my senior year, I started applying to colleges. At the time (1997), there were "Inteflex" medical programs that allowed a person to be accepted into medical school straight from high school contingent on maintaining a 3.75 GPA and passing the entrance interview. The programs are highly competitive and require ACT scores in the 95th percentile, high school GPAs above a 3.8, and a record of extracurricular involvement. Because I was confident that medicine was for me, I was interested in taking this route. I went on about six college interviews and decided on Saint Louis University, which offered me a Dean's scholarship that provided 75% of tuition and room costs for four years of college. Without knowing anyone in St. Louis and with nobody to fill me in on life in the field of medicine, I embarked on my journey to becoming a doctor.

The College Years—August 1997–May 2001

After the rigorous coursework, challenging teachers, and competitive environment in high school, the start of my college career was surprisingly easy. I enrolled as a biology major in the Medical Scholars program, which consisted of 140 well-qualified students who had the desire and credentials in high school to pursue medicine as a career. The program was diverse, with students representing all 50 states. I recall large lecture halls and some rather boring lecturers at the beginning; however, in terms of the coursework, it was similar to high school as far as subject matter and volume. My typical day looked something like this:

Roll out of bed at 7:50 a.m., take classes from 8:00 a.m. until about 2:00 p.m., eat lunch, hit the library until the evening, come back to the dorm, work out, and then hang out with friends. During the weeks leading up to exams, I tended to study until about midnight when the library closed.

Despite the "guarantee" of acceptance to medical school if one maintained a 3.75 GPA, of the 140 students, only about 50 students actually applied to medical school. Some students didn't make the grades and others chose a different career path.

Applying to Med School

Before I knew it, I was entering my junior year of college and it was time for the Medical College Admissions Test (MCAT). MCAT is a standardized test that evaluates potential medical students in areas of biological sciences, physical sciences, and verbal reasoning. The test is about eight hours long, costs $1,000 to take, and is the most important determinant of admission to medical school besides one's grade point average.

I studied for the test along with my regular college course work. I was lucky, however, because as a Medical Scholar with automatic acceptance, there was no minimum MCAT score required for admissions. A few months after the test, it was time to officially apply to medical school. I filled out the 30-page electronic AMCAS application, which included supplemental essays, and asked three professors for letters of recommendation.

I was invited to interview at Saint Louis University School of Medicine. The interview lasted several hours and centered on why I wanted to become a doctor. I explained my desire to help the nation's sick and to use my love of science to accomplish this goal. The interviewers also wanted to get to know me, so we talked about my hobbies and interests as listed on my application, including the prospects for the St. Louis Rams, as well as my family in Michigan. They also asked me where I saw myself in 10 years. I was accepted to the School of Medicine, finished my senior year of college, and before I knew it, I graduated. My journey was just beginning.

CHAPTER 3

My First Year of Medical School—August 2001

THE FIRST DAY OF MEDICAL SCHOOL IS FOREVER etched in my mind. On August 24, 2001, 155 students (40 of them from my Saint Louis University Medical Scholars program) gathered in a cold, dark lecture hall to discuss the outline for our next four years. The lecture hall was massive and framed portraits of past professors adorned the walls. We were all nervous as we looked around at our classmates—students who scored in the 99th percentile on the MCAT, had 3.9 GPAs, were deeply involved in community service and/or medical research, and graduated near the top of their respective colleges.

These were the students who, if they received a score of 98% on a test, immediately thought, "What question did I miss?" If they received an A-, they worried that they were failing and adjusted their study habits accordingly. These were students who were never satisfied with mediocrity, who always wanted to be better than the person next to them. These students lived up to my high school football coach's quote, "Do it better than it ever has been done." This created a competitive, stressful environment, but also a productive one that helped develop high-quality doctors.

On that day, we learned that our first course would be the dreaded anatomy course. We were handed a large syllabus (about eight inches thick and consisting of at least 1,000 pages) and instructed to buy a $500 anatomy atlas that would guide us through our two-month dissection of a human body. (The majority of medical schools begin with this eight-week course, as it is comprehensive and inculcates students into the rigors of the medical school curriculum.)

In high school and college, I was used to other students being less-motivated, less-focused on succeeding academically. I certainly benefitted when my teachers graded using a bell curve. However, now, 155 machine-like, salivating, hard-core students were intently listening to lectures from 8:00 a.m. to noon, going upstairs to the lab to dissect their human cadaver from 12:30 p.m. to 6:00 p.m. and beyond, and then studying all night.

When all the students perform well, the professors are forced to increase the difficulty of test questions—otherwise, all students would get all the questions correct, which wouldn't differentiate an average student from a stellar student. For example, instead of placing a pin with a label on a certain nerve in the cadaver brain and asking, "What nerve is this?" the instructors asked, "If a stroke affected this nerve, what defects would the body have?" The smarter the students, the more complex the questions.

This kind of environment breeds a type of student called a "gunner." Gunners are ultra-competitive, overly ambitious, and will compromise their peer relationships in order to gain recognition and praise from their superiors. They also are obsessed with how others perform.

I remember one gunner in particular. He was the one who asked you how you scored on the test and then responded with, "Oh cool, I got a 99" no matter what you said. He was the first person to arrive in the anatomy dissection lab and the last person to leave. He showed up to 8:00 a.m. lectures at 7:40 a.m. and sat in the first row, raising his hand continually. During breaks between lectures, he introduced himself to the professor and asked complex questions. He packed his lunch, ate it in 10 minutes, and then headed up to the lab for at least six hours. Then, he walked to a fast food restaurant for burgers and fries, which he scarfed down so he could head to the library. He didn't leave the library until midnight, when the lights went dim. He drove home, studied until 2:00 a.m., and then called it a day.

The same ritual was repeated day after day. In the lab, he occasionally walked over to my cadaver to ask how I was doing—verifying along the way that nobody, including me, was overshadowing his achievements. What's funny is that he always acted as though he didn't care, commenting before each exam, "Yeah, I didn't study much. Who knows how I'll do."

I will never forget the smell of formaldehyde in the anatomy lab or the warm slimy feeling on my gloves as I worked to find and isolate nerves and arteries on my cadaver. The human cadaver's organs and nerves never looked like the pictures in the atlas, which was illustrated by a brilliant artist named Frank H. Netter, MD. He drew colorful detailed diagrams of every aspect of human anatomy. The fact that none of my cadavers looked exactly like Dr.

Netter's illustrations reinforced for me the fact that every human being is unique. We do not follow a blueprint. This fact makes the field of medicine very humbling.

Despite the long lectures, peculiar smells, gunners, and lack of sleep, I managed to maintain this daily ritual for the first four weeks of medical school. I often partnered with another student I knew from college. After being in the lab from noon to 6:00 p.m., we went to a white-walled room in the medical school to study until midnight. I lost all contact with the outside world that month. I did not pay attention to the news, sports, anything. That was the culture.

My First Medical School Exam

After four weeks of this monotonous regimen, our first test loomed before us. We began to study even more. Instead of stopping at midnight, we studied until 2:00 a.m. We all began to doubt ourselves. There was so much information to learn from so many resources.

About three days before the first exam, they opened the lab up for 24 hours a day. Sure enough, students were there at 3:00 a.m., trying to soak in every bit of information. I slept for two to three hours the night before the test, thinking I could learn everything. Half the students nervously gathered in a large room to take the written test and the other half gathered in the anatomy lab for the lab section. Four weeks of 15-hour days and four years of college culminated in this moment: my first medical school exam.

My group began in the lab. We walked in to see cadavers with nerves and arteries labeled with needles and small tags. A closer look at the tags and we saw that it wouldn't be a matter of identifying the nerves and arteries. That would be too easy. One tag, positioned on the trigeminal nerve, for example, posed the question, "What artery supplies this nerve?" An alarm sounded every three minutes, prompting us to move to the next station. Three minutes felt like one minute—rushed. After cycling through about 50 stations, we were finished with the lab portion. We went downstairs for the written portion of the exam. Two hours later, I finished my first medical school test and was that much closer to becoming the doctor I'd dreamed of becoming back in seventh grade.

I was only one measly month into a 48-month intense curriculum, but I didn't spend much time thinking about what was to come—which was good.

If I had thought much about the four years of medical school and the three years of residency after that— working 80–100 hours per week with very little sleep—I would've never finished.

A few days after our anatomy exam, our scores were posted outside the lecture hall. Students' hands were shaking as they lined up their finger with their ID number to find their grade. I was happy to see that I had received the second highest score. My study partner was not so happy—his score was average. Of course, an average score among the top students in the nation was nothing to be ashamed of, but he began to doubt himself, wondering if medical school was for him—as did many of my classmates. Some students clearly doubted their abilities. Remember, most of them never even received a B in college. To suddenly get an "average" score was devastating.

However, because of the competitive nature of my fellow students, the majority vowed to study even harder. My study partner persisted and despite his initial doubts, ended up receiving a top 10 score in the class on the next tests. Persistence, grit, and diligence pay off.

Rounding Out the Year

We completed the eight-week anatomy course in October 2001 and then followed an academic curriculum the rest of our first year of medical school. Most of the remaining courses were four weeks in length; the material included pharmacology (how medicines work), physiology (how the human body works), and pathology (the human body viewed from a microscope). Our routine was lectures from 8:00 a.m. to noon, more lectures from 2:00 p.m. to 4:00 p.m., then three to four hours of evening studying. The routine was similar to college, except we had to learn twice the amount of information and the level of competition among my peers was remarkable.

On weekends, I reviewed the lesson plans from the previous week and prepared for the next week of lectures while my non-medical student friends were out having fun or working. I was so busy I really didn't think too much about this, but looking back, I realized I definitely sacrificed a lot by locking myself in that white-walled room to study several hours every day. After that first year, I felt like a well-oiled machine, able to study for hours on end, highlighting my notes and picking out important points that I was confident would pop up on tests. That was the difference between an average student and a top student. Top students could predict what was going to be on the written test.

I used three different highlighters when studying. The blue highlights meant it was certainly going to be tested. The orange highlights meant it was likely to be tested. The yellow highlights meant it was fair game. This system worked very well and I think the strategy really separated the top-notch medical students from the average ones.

And that was the first year—a year of anxiety, vigorous competition, doubts about the future, studying, and the creation of a seasoned veteran capable of handling academic setbacks. I forged ahead despite adversity. I was well on my way to becoming a doctor.

CHAPTER 4

My Second Year of Medical School—August 2002

A S QUICKLY AS THE FIRST YEAR ENDED, my second year began. This year was devoted to learning each body system in sequence. Our first eight weeks were devoted to neurology—everything there was to know about the brain and nerves. Then it was on to cardiology, and so on. The routine was similar. Lectures from 8:00 a.m. to noon, then study until 1:00 a.m. In medical school, I do not recall another student with even a part-time job—there was no time to work. Because every student was an outstanding student, in order to be recognized, or to get a top score, we had to make every point count. Missing just one question on a test could change a score from an Honors grade to a Near Honors grade.

We had a major test about once a month. Most of our tests were graded on a curve, which meant that about 12% of the students received an Honors grade no matter what; 3% received a Near Honors grade; the rest would simply pass or fail. Which takes me to our nephrology exam (the study of the kidneys). For some reason, the professor made the test easier than usual. Or maybe it was difficult, but we all studied extra hard. Consequently 12% of the students received a 99% or better on the test. That meant that a student who received a 98% on the test (obviously a great score) did not Honor the course because only 12% Honor any given test. Rather, that person got a Near Honors score, or a Pass/Fail. My other close competitive friend received a 98% on the exam, yet still did not receive a top score. Thus, he did not receive an Honors. He still cannot believe it and I still joke with him about it to this day.

Not only did we have to excel in the classroom, we also had to prepare for another major standardized test: the United States Medical Licensing Exam (USMLE). The USMLE scores helped determine where we would serve our residency—whether we would go to one of our top choices. The USMLE is a three-part exam.

Step 1, taken after the first year of medical school, evaluates a student's mastery and application of the science concepts that are basic to the practice of medicine. This one-day written exam costs approximately $1,000 to take—not including the cost of preparation books.

Step 2 is taken in the third or fourth year of medical school. This consists of a multiple-choice written exam and a hands-on exam that assesses how students are able to apply their knowledge and skills in interactions with patients, including diagnosing ailments, in a simulated office visit. The application fee for this exam is about $800.

Step 3 of the USMLE is a two-day written exam taken during one's internship (the first year of residency) and leads to a license to practice without supervision. (These USMLE step exams are not the same thing as board exams. Board exams, tests taken after residency, declare a doctor "board certified" in their given field.)

I spent $600 on books to help me prepare for the USMLE exam in June 2003. Anxiety crept in during April and intensified as the academic year ended in May. I arrived at the library—a different library in the community for a change of scenery—at 8:00 a.m. and stayed until 6:00 p.m. every day for the months of May and June. I took the four-hour computerized, multiple-choice test at a testing center in the St. Louis area. This test was actually easier than our regular tests because it was less in depth. Then, it was over and I was entering my third year of medical school.

CHAPTER 5

My Third Year of Medical School—August 2003

URING MY THIRD YEAR OF MEDICAL SCHOOL, I finally had the opportunity to apply the medical knowledge I devoured my first two years to actually affect patient care. I shifted from a machine, memorizing and reciting volumes of information, to a human being capable of using that knowledge to help patients. Instead of driving to the medical school for a lecture every morning, I drove to the hospital to examine patients and do rounds.

Rounds (or the act of rounding) were times in the day when the attending doctor (the senior boss doctor) would meet with all the resident doctors (doctors in training) and the medical students in a conference room and talk about each patient with our list of notes in front of us. The residents and the medical students saw patients early in the morning, examining them from head to toe and asking them questions about how they were feeling. The residents and students then gathered the necessary lab work and their notes from the examinations and met with the attending doctor in the conference room. We discussed what major events happened overnight, went over each patient's lab work and tests, and came up with a tentative plan of care. Then, we left the conference room and walked to each patient's room to talk to and examine each patient separately. This process is called "rounding on patients."

Medical students not only had to possess excellent medical knowledge, they also had to learn great organizational skills. These skills were vital because we had to know everything about 10–12 patients. We also had to develop outstanding bedside manner with patients and work well with a team of doctors. No longer could we be bookworms and still succeed. This year was undoubtedly the most demanding year because we not only had to study for exams at the end of each rotation, we had to wake up very early to

15

round on patients at 5:00 a.m. and stay at the hospital until all the work was done—usually around 8:00 p.m.

The third year was the year to shine because we met professors on rounds who evaluated how well we took care of patients and how well we presented complex information. It was also the most important year for our future because residency programs look at students' third-year grades to help determine who they want in their residency program.

Each medical student was randomly assigned to different specialties his or her third year. The specialties were divided into eight rotations, each focused on a different field of medicine. These rotations included surgery, family medicine, neurology, pediatrics, obstetrics and gynecology, psychiatry, and internal medicine (which includes the specialties of internal medicine such as cardiology, gastroenterology, oncology, and pulmonary).

I was assigned to surgery for my first rotation at the John Cochrane Veterans Administration Medical Center in St. Louis in August 2003. The hospital was associated with Saint Louis University, but was solely for the care of our war veterans. The goal of this eight-week rotation was to become acquainted and involved with patients undergoing surgery.

My First Day on Rotation

I will never forget my first day. Per instructions, I arrived at the hospital workroom at 4:30 a.m., where two other resident doctors were busy recording all the data for the patients they were about to round on. I timidly introduced myself as "Matt the medical student." One resident glared at me, then went straight back to his work. I sat at one of the desks and after about 20 minutes, he said bruskly, "Come with me." I assumed I was going to shadow him on rounds to get an orientation on how things were done. Seconds after leaving the workroom, he received his first page. He scurried to find the nearest phone and called back. The nurse asked that he check on a patient in Room 4032 whose wound looked infected. We hadn't even had a chance to round on our 14 patients yet. I was quickly learning that nothing in medicine is scheduled.

We climbed three flights of stairs and arrived at the patient's room. The patient appeared to have an abscess that was draining pus. My senior resident directed me to get him "some 4 by 4s." I was not sure what he meant, and because I was quite intimidated by his overall terseness, I didn't ask for clarification. Instead, I went to the supply room to try to locate what he wanted. I searched for five minutes and found nothing labeled "4 by 4s." When I returned, I saw that the nurse had given him what he was looking for: white gauze pads that were four inches by four inches. I felt like an idiot! After spending two years studying everything about the human body and learning how every drug and disease process works, I couldn't retrieve a piece of gauze during my first hour of work. The resident looked annoyed, I got over it, and we continued on.

It was now 5:00 a.m. For the next two hours, we visited every patient, meticulously went over their records and lab work on the portable computers, asked them how they were feeling, and performed a physical exam. As we left each patient's room, we grabbed the chart on the wall in the hall and recorded our findings and treatment plan. We began writing a medical note called the SOAP note.

The SOAP note was about one page in length and divided into four components. The first component of the SOAP note was the "S," which stands for "subjective." Here, we recorded how the patient felt and if he or she had any complaints. We also wrote significant things that happened to the patient overnight. For one patient, for example, the resident wrote "s/p leg amputation for diabetes, no fevers overnight, pain controlled with IV Dilaudid. Not passing gas."

The second component was the "O," which stands for "objective." This section included objective findings, such as the vital signs and physical exam findings, using abbreviations. For example, the resident might write, "Temp 37.5, BP 118/72, HR 79, RR 12, pOX 99% RA. Abdomen soft, + BS, heart RRR, lungs CTAB, extremities: no c/c/e, wound c/d/I." (Learning hundreds of abbreviations was daunting.)

The third component of the SOAP note is the "A," which stands for "assessment." This is a brief paragraph that provides an overall assessment and summary of the patient. The resident may write something like, "81 y/o female, POD #1 s/p L BKA, doing well." Basically, an 81-year-old female had an operation one day ago for a left below-the-knee amputation.

The next part is the "P," or "plan." The resident might write, "Continue pain meds, advance diet when bowel sounds are heard, culture if fever."

After signing at the bottom, we moved on to the next of the 13 patients we had that morning. Sometimes we got pages from nurses who had questions about patient care, such as, "Can the patient eat?" or "Patient has a fever. What do you want me to do?" As one can already see, we had to juggle a lot of work, talk to patients, get interrupted by pages, and then resume our previous goal.

This process lasted approximately two hours that first day, which took us to 7:00 a.m.—time for my first surgery, a Whipple pancreaticoduodenectomy. While waiting for the nurses to prep the patient, I changed out of my clothes in the locker room and put on scrubs, then pulled out my book and read about this extensive, complex operation that I had learned about during my first two years of medical school. The operation involved removing the pancreas and surrounding tissue due to pancreatic cancer. It was at least a seven-hour operation because intestines needed to be diverted and blood vessels tied off, in addition to removing the cancerous tissue.

During operations, attending doctors have a habit of "pimping" students or residents—asking difficult medical questions in order to fluster the students. During this particular operation, the doctor asked me, "What artery supplies this part of the pancreas?" Luckily I had stared at the anatomy atlas prior to the operation and correctly responded, "pancreatico-duodenal artery." Over time, students get used to these types of questions and take them in stride, even though they can be very intimidating. This teaches toughness, humility, and perseverance.

The operation was over at 2:00 p.m. The resident, who was also in the operating room, looked at his pager and saw that he had to respond to 10 pages he received during the operation. We grabbed some granola bars for a quick snack, then worked our way back up to the workroom.

We had done our morning rounds and completed a major surgery all before 3:00 p.m. Unfortunately, the day had only begun. Back up in the workroom, the other resident was getting slammed with consults—requests by other doctors or the Emergency Room (ER) to see a patient. We had three of these consults to see, all in the ER. One consult was with regard to a large abscess on the back of a man's neck that we needed to drain. This involved gathering some numbing medicine, cleaning the area of the skin, injecting a needle with medicine directly into the abscess, making a two-inch incision, and watching the pus drain out. We packed the cavity with gauze to allow it to heal. This was a rewarding experience because the patient felt much better. The smell that permeated the room after we opened that abscess is one I will never forget.

We answered more pages, completed more consults, and ended the day at around 8:00 p.m. I drove home, feeling buzzed due to the fact that I had been on the go since 4:30 a.m. I ate some Ramen noodles and set my alarm to 3:30 a.m. As I lay in bed that night, I panicked a bit. Would I be able to keep up this workload in addition to studying for the next step of the USMLE? When would I study if I only got three days off that month? Suddenly, it was 3:30 a.m., the alarm was beeping, and a new day began.

This routine continued for eight weeks, but each day was very different and the days flew by. Some days were spent in the operating room; on other days we saw consult after consult. But the days always began the same way: morning rounds from 5:00 a.m. to 7:00 a.m. and an operation from 7:00 a.m. until at least noon. I stayed overnight at the hospital every fourth night, then stayed the following day until at least 2:00 p.m. I was working about 90 hours per week, and cherished the three days off I had each month. I was able to study for the surgery shelf exam during the 20 minutes I waited for patients to prep in the operating room and during my three days off. (A shelf exam is yet another six-hour standardized multiple-choice test taken after each rotation during the third year of medical school. This test is in addition to tests I have mentioned previously.)

During the remainder of my third year, I rotated through the other fields of medicine. As the weeks passed, I gained more and more responsibility. Eventually, I was able to round on patients in the mornings independently, report my findings to the resident, and write the SOAP notes myself. I realized that what makes our days long are the small things that seem straightforward when writing about them, but actually take much longer in real time. For example, I had to write out the reason for a patient's CAT scan and fax it to the appropriate person in the radiology suite. If the person in radiology didn't receive the fax, I had to re-fax it, which seemed to happen half the time.

The follow-up required for tasks such as these ate up a large part of the day. We had to put in IVs for patients who were difficult, order lab studies or radiology studies, and respond to "codes," which are emergency situations when patients become unresponsive due to heart or lung problems in the hospital. These codes could take an hour or two to resolve.

My Other Rotations

Other rotations were structured differently than my surgery block. For example, during my eight-week pediatrics rotation, I pre-rounded from 6:00 a.m. to 8:00 a.m., meaning I rounded by myself before rounding with the attending doctor. During pre-rounding, I gathered all the laboratory and radiology information for each patient, talked to my 12 or so patients, examined them room by room, wrote the SOAP notes, and prepared to present my findings to the attending doctor. I had to pace myself to ensure I finished in two hours. Often, the radiology studies were not in the computer, so I walked to the radiology department and tried to find the study myself. This could have be a 20–30-minute detour, depending on how quickly I could find the right person. Sometimes families arrived just as I finished with a patient, so I had to re-explain the treatment plan.

At 8:00 a.m., the attending physician arrived at the hospital and we rounded on the patients in their respective rooms. Outside the room, I presented my findings to the residents, other students on the rotation, and the attending doctor. He usually pimped me and asked for the results of the radiology and laboratory studies. We found a nearby computer and looked at the radiology images ourselves. As a gunner (yes, I admit it), I looked up scientific articles that pertained to my patient and presented them on rounds. I presented the physical exam findings and then summarized what I thought was best for the patient in terms of an assessment and plan. The attending doctor added his words of wisdom before we walked into the patient's room, talked with the patient and his or her family members, and came up with a plan of action. This was the process for all the patients we had that day, which included up to 20 patients. (I had 10 patients and my fellow medical student had another 10 patients.)

After rounds, which usually lasted from 8:00 a.m. to noon, we broke for an hour-long learning lecture called morning report. This meeting was usually led by a resident who was prepared to present a patient's admission. We talked about a patient in detail and presented all the available literature in terms of diagnosis and treatment of that patient. Other residents on the floors attended as well, so the room was filled with about 30 residents, medical students, and attending doctors. If we were lucky, subs or pizza were offered during morning report. After morning report, we answered all the pages we got during that hour-long learning experience. Then, we ordered our radiology tests and blood tests, interpreted findings, and accepted new patients to admit.

Let me clarify what admitting a patient entails. When a patient comes into the ER for a specific complaint, the ER doctor evaluates the patient and determines if that patient can be sent home or should be admitted to the hospital. If he or she determines the patient should be admitted, the ER doctor calls the admitting team of doctors and explains the reason for admission. The admitting team then sees the patient and writes orders for that patient. The admitting doctor writes a history and physical exam, which is similar to a SOAP note, but more encompassing. This note includes the family history, social history, and other medical/surgical problems the patient has. The patient is transferred to the hospital floor and we see him or her again in the morning.

The process of admitting patients and ordering tests continued until about 6:00 p.m., when another admitting team took over. Again, this process *seems* to be streamlined, but it's more complicated than it appears. For example, if I wanted a simple blood test, I wrote the order in the chart and personally notified the nurse. Many times, the nurses did not see the order or the clerk who processes the order did not see it or entered it incorrectly. So I needed to follow up frequently to make sure it was done correctly. Sometimes, I got so frustrated that I drew the blood myself in between admitting patients, answering multiple pages, and following up other patients' tests.

Patients need to go home eventually, and that took time as well. Discharging a patient involved writing a six- or seven-page report explaining why the patient was admitted, what treatment was provided during the hospital stay, and what the future plan of care should be. After all was said and done, I usually left the hospital at 9:00 p.m. or so, went home, got something to eat, and went to bed, knowing I'd be back again to round at 6:00 a.m. Time flew by because we were always so busy and three days seemed like one long day.

I did other rotations during my third year as well, including my eight-week obstetrics and gynecology block in January and February. I learned how to deliver babies, which was interesting. The actual delivery of the baby was the easy part. I recall a very moody resident during that rotation who wanted all the information and all the patients ready by 5:00 each morning—which meant I had to come in at 3:30 a.m.

I ended my third year of medical school with the 12-week internal medicine rotation. This field most closely resembled our medical school studies, as we could apply the concepts we learned in the variety of subject areas we studied during our second year. For example, if we saw a patient who had a heart attack and then went into kidney failure, we could apply concepts we learned during our kidney rotation and cardiology rotation to help that patient.

I enjoyed this rotation because it required detective work—answers were not always apparent. For example, I admitted a patient who exhibited shortness of breath. After ruling out the common causes associated with the heart and lungs, I needed to look further and consider less-common causes. That's when the detective work comes in. I asked the patient more questions about his social history and learned that he was a farmer. There is a condition called hypersensitivity pneumonitis—an allergic reaction in the lung caused by moldy hay. After further tests, our team determined this was the most likely diagnosis.

Many students put forth more effort on this rotation because a common path in medical school is to do internal medicine in residency. Therefore, it was important to receive excellent reviews from one's attending doctors and perform well on the internal medicine shelf exam after the rotation.

On this rotation, we were responsible for about six patients. On a typical day during my internal medicine rotation, I arrived at the hospital at 6:00 a.m., pre-rounded on my six patients, and gathered all the radiology, lab work, and notes from nurses and the doctor on call the previous night. I then walked to each room, examined each patient, asked him or her pertinent questions, answered the patient's family's questions, and then determined what needed to be done to get them discharged. This process was intense because most patients had multiple medical problems and took several medications—usually at least 10, and sometimes more than 30. So I had to make sure everything was in order. As with the other rotations, I had to complete my SOAP notes, answer pages, draw blood if necessary, round with the attending doctor, attend the morning report, order lab and radiology tests, admit new patients, and work on discharging patients.

Discharging patients was a huge task. Many of these patients were very sick, many were elderly and could barely talk or hear, let alone walk out of a hospital by themselves. We had to review each medication they were on (usually more than 15) and coordinate where they were going when they left the hospital. Some patients went to a nursing home, others to a rehab facility. Although social workers usually were the ones who arranged where the patient was going upon discharge, sometimes we called the facilities ourselves. Ideally, the patient went home with the family, but many patients had no family in the area or were too sick to go home.

All the while, we were receiving page after page from nurses or the lab asking relatively minor questions or notifying us that something was not inputted correctly. The high rate of needless pages tested our patience and inhibited our ability to multitask. For example, I was at the hospital bedside counseling a family of seven about a new diagnosis of lung cancer. I received a STAT page, which signaled an emergency. I excused myself from the room in mid-conversation, found an unoccupied phone in the hallway and called the number back. The clerk who answered simply wanted to know if a patient could have something to eat. I provided a terse "yes," then started back to the waiting family.

Of course, in the meantime, I received another STAT page about a code, meaning a patient's heart or lungs stopped functioning. I ran to the room to help the residents, nurses, and clerks stabilize the patient. One resident performed chest compressions, another placed a breathing tube, another tried get a better arterial line to administer strong medications, and another recorded times because every second counts. Someone gathered the correct meds, another administered the meds, and another ran the blood tests to the lab. The senior resident continually shouted out orders during our attempt to revive the patient. It was the epitome of organized chaos. Unfortunately, after 20 minutes of doing everything humanly possible to revive this patient, we could never restore his pulse. The code was complete, the family was notified, and we carried on with our day.

One hour had elapsed since I left the initial patient's room. I went back in, apologized to the family, and resumed my emotional conversation about a terminal cancer—just after I observed another patient die. Talk about a 20-something medical student taking on some very important roles. Now, I was back to square one after an hour delay. These delays (pages) were very common, which made my job harder than meets the eye. As you can see, we had to multitask and be able to filter out important versus unimportant pages all while trying to complete our daily tasks.

When on call, we continued this routine throughout the night with little or no sleep. We also covered the patients whose doctors were not on call. Because we were now covering other doctors' patients from 6:00 p.m. to 7:00 a.m., we got triple the number of pages. We typically admitted 5 new patients overnight. Because these patients were admitted at all hours, we were always up, answering calls about the 40 patients we were covering, admitting a new patient, or typing admission notes on the patients. We also responded to codes, did complex procedures like inserting a catheter into someone's large neck vein, or went down to radiology to read a CAT scan or MRI. There was always something, which made time fly by, but it also left us with no sleep.

By the time 8:00 a.m. came around again, we were ready to round. So on hour number 24, we were presenting complex patients to our attending doctor, answering pimp questions, answering pages, and writing our SOAP notes with the hope of leaving the hospital by 1:00 p.m. In reality, we left at around 3:00 p.m. I went home, ate something, slept from 5:00 p.m. to 8:00 p.m., woke up for dinner, then slept again until 5:00 a.m. to go to the hospital. They say whatever doesn't break you makes you stronger. I definitely developed thick skin that would prepare me for the even longer hours of residency in two years.

After this intense 12-week rotation in internal medicine, I realized I really did enjoy it. I loved seeing patients who were sick with multiple problems and trying to make them better. I felt like a detective trying to solve a puzzle, with labs, x-rays, and my stethoscope as my tools. I ended my third year with the idea that I could train in internal medicine and have the option to specialize afterward. I did well on the internal medicine shelf exam because when I had some time here and there during my call nights, I read and caught up on my studies. I was beginning to realize my dreams of becoming a doctor. But dreams materialize slowly.

Side Note: A Memorable Night—May 2004

As medical students, we tried to make the most of our three or four nights off per month during our third-year rotations. Most nights, we studied to catch up on the rotation exam. Other nights, though, we simply needed a break. One night, my friend Javier and I went out to a bar in St. Louis, about 15 minutes from the hospital. We were not big on dancing, but did enjoy hanging out and taking in the scenery. At around 2:00 a.m., I noticed two girls dancing together, having a good time. I decided to walk up to one of them and start dancing with her. We danced until the club closed, then I suggested that we all go to a local breakfast joint to chat some. Javier was tired and declined, so I hitched a ride with Jackie and Mary to the diner, where we talked over eggs and juice for another few hours. At 5:00 a.m., we left the restaurant, they dropped me off at my apartment, and I waved goodbye to Jackie, my future wife.

CHAPTER 6

My Fourth Year of Medical School—July 2004

MY FOURTH YEAR OF MEDICAL SCHOOL allowed me to get more specific about what I wanted in a career. I did several months of elective rotations; options included dermatology, ophthalmology, emergency medicine, radiology, or specialties in medicine, such as cardiology or gastroenterology. It also gave me an opportunity to train at a different center so I could experience other health systems. These were called externships. I applied to do an externship at Beth Israel Hospital in Boston, which is a Harvard-affiliated hospital. I was accepted and planned to do the externship in November 2004, during my fourth year of medical school.

I began my fourth year with emergency medicine. The rapid diagnosis and treatment of sick patients prompted me to sign up for this elective. It was also procedure-oriented, so I had the opportunity to place chest tubes in patients who had motor vehicle accidents or place breathing tubes in patients who could not breathe on their own. Initially, I thought the workload would be less because my hours were based on shifts rather than a grueling on-call schedule. However, after a month, I realized the work is simply different, not necessarily easier. A continuous stream of trauma patients arrive, and they often are actively bleeding or have life-threatening issues. The ER doctor is always under pressure to make split-second decisions. But, I liked the opportunity to fix the problem and send patients home. Maybe it was a patient with a large skin laceration that I stitched up or a patient with a separated shoulder that I put back in place.

Unfortunately, many patients treat the ER not as an emergency center for emergencies, but rather as a primary care office. They come in with requests for medication refills or exacerbations of medical problems that an office doctor should be able to see. Many patients who are being treated for chronic pain use the ER as a place to get IV pain medications, which certainly can be provided as an outpatient service. Patients often are intoxicated, which can make for a hostile environment. Nurses and doctors are cursed at or belittled as entitled patients demand pain medications or food. I could not see spending my career as an ER doctor.

One patient in the ER helped me decide what area I did want to pursue, however. This 52-year-old woman came into the ER for neck pain. After taking a detailed history and doing a physical exam, I realized that she could have meningitis. I got approval from the attending ER doctor to perform a lumbar puncture, which entailed inserting a large needle into the spinal space in her spine and removing a small amount of spinal fluid. Based on a lab analysis of the fluid, I determined it likely was meningitis, and called the admitting doctor to admit her to the hospital. When I hung up, I realized that my interaction with this patient was done; I would not know her final outcome. The lack of follow-up and inability to figure out final solutions dissuaded me from pursuing a career in the ER. I also tended to enjoy the complex workups of patients with rare diseases. ER medicine is great for those who enjoy trauma and surgery, but I leaned more toward internal medicine.

My Introduction to Gastroenterology

My second elective during my fourth year was gastroenterology, a specialty of internal medicine. Little did I know at the time that this was the field I would fall in love with. This specialty involved treating diseases of the gastrointestinal tract and liver. Gastroenterology/Hepatology is a three-year fellowship after completion of a three-year internal medicine residency. Other fellowships include cardiology, nephrology, pulmonary, critical care, and oncology.

I began the rotation observing the gastroenterology fellows (doctors who have completed residency and are now specializing further) perform endoscopies. I was in awe of the sophistication of these endoscopes. The doctors could see polyps that were only 2 millimeters in size! The way the fellow maneuvered the endoscope reminded me of a fun video game—except that he was saving someone's life. I watched these scopes beyond my expected hours just because each one was so different. To be able to visualize inside someone's body with that resolution was amazing.

As I learned other aspects of gastroenterology and hepatology, I became even more interested. Gastroenterologists see patients who need to have a procedure done immediately, as well as patients who have more long-term, chronic conditions such as Crohn's disease or celiac disease, which means a doctor-patient relationship can develop. There are opportunities to consider the different causes of a disease, such as liver disease, and use medical knowledge and other tools to figure it out. Finally, this field allowed me to perform procedures to save lives, such as colonoscopies, which remove precancerous polyps.

So during the latter half of this month-long rotation, I knew this was what I wanted in a career: a specialist who deals with diseases of the bowel, pancreas, and liver—a gastroenterologist. I felt this field offered a great deal of variety. I could perform high-tech procedures to prevent cancer in my patients. I could develop patient-doctor relationships in the office with those patients who had chronic conditions such as Crohn's disease or irritable bowel syndrome. And I could also do urgent, adrenaline-pumping procedures. It was a good mix of everything.

Applying for Residency Programs

In August, it was time to begin applying to various residency programs. That meant months of filling out application forms, getting letters of recommendation, and traveling to programs around the United States for interviews. Medical students are granted an interview based on merit; students may go on as many as 15 interviews. After all interviews for the thousands of medical students are completed between October and the end of January, the medical students and the residency programs rank each other to form a rank list.

On Match Day, a computer program matches the medical students' top choices with the residency programs' top choices. All students gather in an auditorium and are handed a letter that indicates which residency accepted them and where they would be spending the next three to six years of their life. For example, if a medical student ranks a program first and a residency program ranks that person in the top 25, that person would "match" and thus enroll in that residency program. If that student ranked a program high, but the program did not think highly of the medical student, the student would get bumped down to his or her second choice, and so on, until the student reached the bottom of his or her rank list.

I began to prepare my electronic application in August 2004 by gathering a variety of items. I had to get three letters of recommendation from attending doctors who would vouch for my competence, describing my work ethic, intelligence, perseverance, and interactions with patients. During my nights away from the hospital, I wrote a personal one-page statement about why I wanted to be at a particular residency program. I gathered the extensive information necessary to fill out the 30-page application. This form asked about demographics, grades in medical school, community service, scores on USMLE exams, etc. After this month-long process I submitted my 15 applications—along with the $100 fee per application. As I hit the submit button, I realized that I also had to cover the expense of traveling to each program for the interviews. That meant taking out a $4,000 loan.

In November, I had the opportunity to do an externship. Because my college roommate lived in Boston and attended MIT, and because Beth Israel had a strong internal medicine program, I applied to do a month-long externship there. They accepted me and I was able to stay at my friend's apartment and use the subway system for transportation to cut costs. I read the book *The House of God* prior to going to Boston, which made the experience that much more interesting. This funny satirical first-hand account of the rigors and mishaps of medicine was set at Beth Israel, and some of the characters in the book were doctors there! I learned a lot from the externship about adjusting to different styles of medicine, and my 80-hour work weeks helped me prepare for the real rigors of internal medicine residency.

Interviewing for Residency

After arriving back in St. Louis at the end of November, I was ready to begin interviewing for residency spots while taking other elective courses. I tried to take lighter rotations these months so I would have the chance to go on the interviews *and* prepare for USMLE Step 2. This test is similar to the USMLE Step 1, but more clinical, as we now took care of patients. I registered for the USMLE Step 2 in November and submitted my $800 fee for this test. In addition, we had to take a second part of the Step 2 called the "CS" or Clinical Skills part. This required us to fly to a larger city (in my case, Chicago) to take part in role-playing interviews on patients to prove that we could solve dilemmas and treat patients with respect. Unfortunately, this cost another $800 plus the cost of flight and hotel, which added another $400— quite a bit for a person with no income. Nevertheless, I spent many nights preparing for this test when I was not interviewing or doing my electives.

We still worked weekends and weekdays, so we had to be creative about when and how we got to these interviews. We also had to be cost-conscious. I remember carpooling with a friend to interview at the Mayo Clinic in Rochester, Minnesota. The roads were slick, but the flight costs were prohibitive. We left in the evening after work, taking turns driving, interviewed for a day, and then turned right around so we could be back at the hospital the following day.

The night before the interview, we typically met with the current residents at a restaurant and asked them personal questions about how they liked the program and got to know some of their personalities. I particularly remember the night of my University of Michigan program interview. Jackie, then my fiancée, and I drove in from St. Louis on a snowy evening and stayed at my parents' home. The next afternoon, I drove to Ann Arbor to attend the dinner with the residents. We actually arrived a few hours early because I was obsessed about being early for events such as this. We went to a local restaurant to have a drink and were pleasantly surprised by happy hour tacos and other snacks. Then we strolled out and began to look for the restaurant designated for our interview dinner: Grizzly Peak.

I expected 4-6 residents to show up for a low-key meal, as had been the case in previous interviews. Michigan, however, really did it up! We walked into the restaurant and at least 30 residents were there drinking microbrews. We sat down at a table and they immediately starting talking about life in Ann Arbor and how much they enjoyed themselves. I ended up staying at this interview dinner for a few hours and really got to know some of the residents. I felt I could relate to them, as we all had similar interests, such as sports, which showed they had a pretty well-rounded life and that they tried to do something of quality with their "free time." There was also a good mix of those who were married with families and those who were single. We left that evening with a good impression and felt that we "clicked" with several of the residents.

The actual interviews usually consisted of meeting with three to four faculty at the residency program. They asked why we wanted to be there, what our strengths/weaknesses were, etc. We toured the hospital, attended the morning reports with the residents, and then asked questions. During the interview day in Michigan, I was able to meet all the residents and faculty at a professional level. The program was open about allowing us to interact with them during the interview. Other programs were more restrictive and did not allow as much interaction, which raised red flags for me. In addition, other programs didn't have the full participation that Michigan offered. For example, for one interview, I flew into New York the night before my interview and was told to meet at a sushi restaurant in Manhattan. Other candidates arrived at the restaurant, but it wasn't until much later that one resident arrived, very disheveled and obviously uninterested in talking about the program. However, during my interview at the University of Michigan, I noted that the residents were engaged and excited about where they trained.

In addition, they had one of the largest gastroenterology divisions in the nation with many leaders in the field. I was able to talk with a few of them during the interview day and was impressed by their hard-working, yet friendly attitudes.

The months of January through March seemed to fly by. I was taking various elective courses, such as a radiology reading elective and an elective to learn how to read EKGs better. Knowing I likely would not see them after that year, I tried to spend more time with friends I had made during those four years. In addition to being separated by miles, we would be toiling under 80–100-hour work weeks, so our bond would unfortunately be lost. And in the back of our minds, we knew this.

Little did I know that at that point in my life, the journey was still in its early stages. I would still have to endure a taxing three years of residency. Sometimes, being naïve is beneficial. By taking each day at a time, rather than looking collectively at such a long, hard, competitive road, I was able to reach my daily goals. And because I was so busy, weeks passed by like days, hours like minutes.

So, during this time, we enjoyed going to the local bars, having a few beers, and reminiscing about our early years of medical school, when we freaked out about even passing medical school. We joked about my friend who thought he was going to fail out, yet ended up doing particularly well. We talked about the medical students who were near the bottom of the class and needed remedial support from our anatomy professor. Or we joked about the gunners who refused to leave the library and studied like a machine day in and day out. We realized we were chiseled veterans, having spent hundreds of hours in the hospital treating patients. We went from not knowing what a piece of gauze was to being called on to handle life-threatening medical diseases. We were finally able to use the medical knowledge we learned during the first two years of medical school and apply it to real patients. Soon, we would be called doctors.

In February, I took my USMLE Step 2 exam—another 8-hour exam that was multiple choice. It was tiring, but because we are so used to studying for 15 hours per day for tests, this 8-hour exam really was just another day. After the written portion of Step 2, I had to catch a flight to take the oral portion of the exam in Chicago. This involved me being on camera and diagnosing fake patients with diseases based on what they told me and what their physical exam turned out to be. This was over before I knew it, and I was down yet another $1,600 for the cost of the test, flight, and hotel.

When I finished my 12 interviews, I was ready to rank the programs based on quality of program, location, reputation, rigor of work, and potential for the future in my field of interest, which was gastroenterology. I contemplated for hours on end about the pros and cons of each program and how to rank them. I got input from my parents and from Jackie about where we would likely end up. After much discussion, including going on medical forums, Jackie and I decided the University of Michigan was the best fit for us. The people really made the difference and the location near my family in Michigan helped. In addition, it had a large gastroenterology division, which would allow me to do research to promote my interest in the field. The division had a reputation as having a group of very hard-working residents who were challenged, but were proud of their institution. Also, I "bled blue" as a child, and coming back to support the Michigan Wolverines community was very appealing!

I also considered programs such as Beth Israel in Boston, where I spent the month doing an externship, and the University of Chicago, where the program was considerably smaller. After much thought, I opened up the electronic rank list and ranked each program 1–12 and hit "submit."

CHAPTER 7

Match Day—March 18, 2005

O N MARCH 18, 2005, ALL THE MEDICAL STUDENTS in the nation gathered at their respective schools to find out where they would be spending the next three to six years of their lives. There is a range because all programs have different training lengths. For example, internal medicine is three years, general surgery is five years, and neurosurgery is six years.

This was the day when four hard, competitive years were sealed up in a white envelope, ready to change one's life forever. Our school rented out a hall 15 minutes from the medical school for this event. Friends and family gathered with us. Everyone was nervous, yet relieved that this day had finally come. Remember, the goal was a match. If a student loved a residency program, but that love was not reciprocated by the residency program, that student would not match. If a program really wanted a student, but that student didn't rank the program highly, that student would not match at that particular program. The goal was to match the student's highest-ranked program with the program's highest-ranked students.

After about an hour of mingling and eating appetizers, our medical school dean took his place, called each student to the front, and handed us each a white envelope. Inside that envelope was the answer to the question about where we would be spending the next several years. I opened my envelope with the same emotion I remember opening up Christmas presents when I was younger. I was elated when I saw "University of Michigan-Ann Arbor, Internal Medicine."

The residency program began in the middle of June, so at the end of March, it was time to start preparing for relocation. We were trying to be responsible financially, despite having $200,000 in school loans, not to mention the other hefty costs, including my medical school exams ($5,000), living expenses ($12,000/year), application fees/interview costs ($4,000), and relocation costs ($5,000). Unfortunately, loans were not available to cover some of these expenses, so my credit card balance was exceedingly high with an unfavorable interest rate.

In medical school, we didn't have time to earn money with a regular job. We were busy working in the hospital 80 hours per week and studying for exams in our "spare time." If we did not have the luxury of parental support, every expense during those four years was paid for by loan or by credit card, including underwear, toothpaste, rent, and food on top of moving and expensive medical exams with money that we didn't have! I still feel this is unfair as the programs expected us to have this money available for interviews and exams even though they knew we had no income in medical school. And these exams were not cheap! Many exams cost at least $1,000 to take.

Thankfully, our medical school offered a $10,000 "relocation loan" with a 5% interest rate, which helped immensely. Jackie and I thought about the benefits of buying a home versus renting. At the time, in April 2005, homes were appreciating at a rate of 15% per year with no signs of slowing down. In addition, "doctor's loans" allowed future resident physicians to obtain a home mortgage without a down payment. Certain banks offered these at attractive rates of around 5.5%.

Because I was taught that a home was an investment and that renting was simply "throwing money away," we decided to take out yet another loan for our first home together in Ann Arbor, Michigan. We were pre-approved for around $230,000 despite having over $200,000 in debt and no history of income. It still amazes me that banks allowed this, as our incomes in residency were no more than $40,000/year, usually in the $37,000 range. Yet, they must've thought that a frugal doctor who had a steady job as a resident physician could afford to pay off a loan, as they were used to large loan payoffs!

All the medical students met in a lecture hall during that spring so a financial advisor could talk to us about loans and loan consolidation. I had college as well as medical school debt, and remember the advisor talking about rolling all these loans into one and getting a fixed interest rate—2.85% at that time—so I decided that's what I would do. I had $196,000 in loans in addition to other private loans and relocation loans. That does not even take into account the large sums of high-interest credit card debt. After this session, most of us just shook our heads. We were so used to letting the debt rack up that we didn't worry about these large numbers. We didn't have time to worry—we had patients to care for and rigorous exams to pass.

From the end of March through April 2005, I drove to Ann Arbor several times to look at homes. I still had my electives to do as well as review material to prepare for residency. I often had to travel alone, as Jackie was working on her Ph.D. We finally decided on a condominium. It was close to the hospital (nine-minute commute), close to Michigan stadium (huge Wolverine fan), and was in a nice neighborhood. It needed some work—built in 1979—but I fell for the location. After getting all our finances in order, we closed on our first condominium together on May 17, 2005 for $176,500.

Because we had no money for closing costs, I negotiated to have our $5,000 closing costs rolled into the mortgage, making our actual loan $181,500. Despite our effort to be fiscally responsible, our overall debt load swelled to more than $450,000. But we were happy and sure that the value of the condo would appreciate, as the housing market was healthy in 2005. We used our $10,000 relocation loan to move both our cars and the small amount of clothes and furniture. We also used some of this loan to refurbish the floors and carpet in the condo to make it suitable for living.

Before we knew it, it was June and the next big journey was about to begin. We had gotten married with a small reception among close friends and were excited to continue our life together in Ann Arbor. Jackie enrolled in a Ph.D. program at Wayne State University and worked part time at the University of Michigan and Washtenaw Community College to help pay some bills.

I attended a couple of orientation events such as picnics, where I met my future co-residents. These men and women were to become my fellow warriors. The people I met during orientation were some of the most talented individuals I have ever come across. Most came from very prestigious programs and oozed confidence. Little did we know that our confidence would be tested during the most strenuous time of our lives: our internship. We call the three-year program "residency," but the first year is technically called "internship." I would do one year of internship, followed by two years of residency for a total of three years of training in internal medicine—tested to the point of wanting to break down and cry, crawl into a corner of the hospital, and hope to never be found.

CHAPTER 8

My Internship (Residency)— June 2005–June 2006

J UNE 24, 2005. I HAD COMPLETED MEDICAL SCHOOL and earned my MD degree. The orientation picnics were over. The happiness of completing medical school and earning that MD degree was over. The joy of achieving that medical doctorate suddenly means we have to use this degree to treat patients.

Residency had officially begun: three years of intense physical, emotional, and mental work that will never be replicated. This first day was akin to being thrown into an ocean and forced to sink or swim. One would think you would be eased into the position, starting with orientation and shadowing of a fellow physician. That wasn't the case. We went from taking care of 6 patients in medical school under close supervision, to caring for 12 patients with us calling the shots. It was as if the MD was an enchantment of infallibility, a degree that made me intellectually superior, emotionally strong, and physically able to perform well without sleep. We now had to have all the answers to anyone throwing questions at us—nurses, patients, colleagues, families.

I met with the intern—a second-year resident who was on service from the previous month—to get a sign out, a list of the 12 patients she was taking care of, along with their medical history, lab and radiology studies, and plans of care. Because she was leaving the general medicine rotation and I was starting, she briefly filled me in about each patient and the goal of care. We sat in our doctor "workrooms," which were centrally located to the patient rooms. Patient names were scribbled on dry erase boards and old Wendy's fast food containers were scattered around the rooms.

The sign-out process lasted about 15 minutes. An example of a sign out is as follows: "Patient Smith, an 88 y/o male who was admitted with shortness of breath and anemia. He was found to have a pulmonary embolism, is now on heparin, and plans on getting an IVC filter. He had some bleeding per rectum as well. He also has stage III heart failure. Plan: workup anemia and bleeding, optimize cardiac meds, start Coumadin, and discharge when stable." This is a "brief" summary of one patient out of the 12 we would be taking care of. That care involved concentrating on several different problems, from assessing his bleeding to managing his heart, lungs, and blood clots. It involved making sure all his labs were done, radiology tests were ordered, the family was informed, and he had a place to be discharged to when he left the hospital.

Remember, for interns, nothing is simple. For example, I wanted to talk to Mr. Smith about his heart failure symptoms. Unfortunately, it seemed that every time I went to his room, he was down in a radiology suite getting a test done, so I would have to come back later. When I did catch him in his room and was able to spend 15 minutes talking with him, five family members walked in as I was walking out. Consequently, I spent another 15 minutes repeating the conversation I had just had with Mr. Smith.

Sometimes I had to communicate with a patient who was confused and who had no social support. I would look up contact information for and call the next of kin or call the social worker to help me with the communication problems. Another issue centered on getting a successful blood draw in order to analyze the labs. Many times, nurses were unable to draw blood due to blown out or thin veins. So in addition to interpreting and taking action based on the results of labs, we sometimes had to think of ways to draw the blood ourselves.

Another common issue concerned radiology. Let's say I wanted to order an IVC filter for Mr. Smith to protect his lung from future blood clots. If I wrote the order and personally faxed it to radiology, there was a good chance they would not receive the fax. In that case, I had to verify everything and resend the order. The frustrating part was that if radiology didn't receive the order, it simply would not happen. Therefore, I had to do follow-up work to ensure they received the order.

In the end, all the responsibility was with the resident physicians. This type of extra work added hours to our days. We had to multitask even more, yet remain steadfast to ensuring our patients' health. One could argue this made us stronger, but it also aged us tremendously.

Which brings me back to my first day of internship. I received the sign out from the newly minted second-year resident. Then, I began the task of pre-rounding from 6:00 a.m. to 8:00 a.m. Afterwards, I rounded with the attending staff until noon. I attended morning report and then completed the work for the day: ordering lab studies, following up those labs, ordering radiology studies, and discharging patients from the hospital.

Since it was my first day, however, everything took longer than expected. I was still new to the computer systems and did not know where anything was located or how to contact the correct people. For example, a nurse would ask us about supplementing a patient's potassium, yet we didn't yet know how to write that order. We didn't even know how to call the nurse back! Thus, my co-intern John and I had a long first day, from 6:30 a.m. until 9:00 p.m. We spent time learning how to order a basic chest x-ray and how to answer pages from nurses, in addition to learning everything we could about the 12 patients we each inherited. I remember walking out with him that first day, thinking, "Oh my God, we survived one day, but we have three years of this." And that was not even our call night.

First Call Night of Internship—June 27, 2005

It was my third day of internship, which for me meant my first call day. Based on the framework of our program of 34 residents per class (three classes total, as we have three years of residency), we would be on call every fourth night when we were on "service months." Service months are months when we care for patients who are physically in the hospital. It can include work we do on the cancer floors (wards), pulmonary floors, cardiology floors, gastroenterology floors, intensive care unit, or general medicine floors.

As I sat home the night before my first call, I assured Jackie that we would get through this together. As we went for our evening walk that night, I remember thinking, "I will leave our home at 5:50 a.m., not see the light of day, work all night, and come home the next day at 3:00 p.m. Thirty-three hours of straight work. And I will do this every fourth night for a year."

Even though I did this in medical school during my third and fourth years, this was different because we now had full responsibility for our patients. We did not have residents to look to; we were the residents. We did have our attending physicians, but these doctors left after 5:00 p.m. and we were on our own after that. We, all of sudden, were the resident physicians, the ones trained to care for our nation's sick and prolong their lives. We were the ones who had to know all the answers when nurses or lab technicians or patients or family members asked us questions. If we didn't know, we had to find out. I was a student one day and a doctor the next.

On my first call day, I woke up at 5:15 a.m., as I did most days as a student. Because I was able to shorten my commute to nine minutes by taking side streets, I was in the hospital by 5:50 a.m. I first had to track down the covering resident to get my sign out, as he was on call the previous night. I found out he was in the ER evaluating a patient, and after five wrong turns, I eventually made it there. When he had a second, he quickly scrolled through his multi-page lists of patients, as he had covered five doctors the previous night—which meant he was covering 60 patients in addition to his own, not including the new patients he admitted that night.

He pulled out my 12 patients and went through them one by one, referring to his written notes for each. One patient actually coded and passed away that night. She was sick with a rare vasculitis of her lungs, and developed respiratory arrest from blood pooling in her lungs. Another patient had severe pain all night and needed extra doses of pain meds. Another patient had his IV fall out and needed to have a more permanent line placed. One patient's CAT scan results had been phoned in to the covering doctor and showed a new liver cancer.

After I received the information I needed, I headed back up to the sixth floor to pre-round on my patients. This meant gathering information on each patient one by one, stopping by their rooms, performing a physical exam, interviewing them with or without their families, and then coming up with a plan in preparation for rounds with the attending doctor.

This was rather stressful for several reasons:

1. We knew our attending doctor would arrive at 8:00 a.m., so we had to make sure all our work was done by then or we would be considered inefficient.

2. We received multiple pages by nurses, social workers, or radiologists while we were with patients. Leaving the patient's room to answer urgent pages disrupted our workflow. Even something as simple as running out of latex gloves or lubricant could hinder us three to four minutes because we had to leave the patient's room and search for the needed item—which often was locked in a supply room 30 yards down the hall. We had to page a nurse to figure out the code to get into the supply room or track someone down to help us.

3. Some patients were sicker than others, which meant we had to modify when and how we saw the patients, sometimes leaving one patient's room to tend to another higher-priority patient.

4. The page requesting a "doctor draw" meant a nurse could not draw the blood due to difficulty accessing the patient's veins, so the resident had to gather the correct equipment to perform a blood draw, prep the patient, retrieve the correct tubes to send to the lab, fill out the paperwork, then perform the task. This simple page could cost us 15–20 minutes because different tubes were often in a different location than the blood draw kit. Nothing was worse than trying to examine a difficult patient only to get paged in the middle of the process.

During my first call day, I actually got that dreaded "doctor draw" before I even saw my first patient around 6:20 a.m. I walked briskly to the supply room to find a needle, gauze, tubes, and a tourniquet. Of course, all of these respective items were in different areas, which wasted valuable time. I walked back to that patient's room, which was about 30 yards away, and performed this five-minute procedure. Afterwards, I interviewed the patient, recorded his vital signs, and performed a physical exam. I then proceeded to see the other 11 patients, one by one.

The standard was to arrive at the patient's room and open the paper chart hanging outside of the room. If the chart was not there, I had to look for it at the nurses' station or with another doctor. I recorded vital signs, what medications were given, and significant events overnight. I needed to know how many bowel movements the patients had, how much urine they produced, and how much pain they had overnight, among many other things. After scouring the charts, I walked into the room, talked with the patient, performed a physical exam, and then recorded my thoughts. I then made a to-do list on a piece of paper I carried everywhere. Examples might be "Order CT A/P, check c. dif toxin, follow up chest x-ray, check placement." I drew a hollow square next to each item, and then checked the box when I completed the task. This helped me stay organized, as we may have 5–10 to-do items multiplied by 12 patients, totaling 60–120 things to do each day—not to mention other tasks we got paged about or other patients who needed further attention.

At 8 a.m., my attending doctor walked into the resident workroom. Our senior resident paged me and John, my co-intern, to make us aware that the attending doctor had arrived. Once our team was all present, we walked to each patient's room, gave the attending doctor an update, and presented our assessment and plan for the respective patient. He modified our plans, shared his expertise, and asked us questions about the patients. Some attending doctors had reputations for asking very difficult questions in an attempt to stump hard-working residents and keep them humble. For example, my attending doctor asked John, "The bite of a scorpion from what country can cause pancreatitis?" Not only did John have to know that a scorpion bite can cause pancreatitis, he had to know the country. That is a very detailed pimp question.

In addition to this rounding, which lasted until about 10:30 a.m., I received about 10 pages per hour with questions nurses had about patients, including urgent ones, which meant we had to interrupt our discussions with our fellow doctors to answer them. If a family member was out of the room getting breakfast, we often returned to the room to talk to the family for an extra 15–20 minutes. If a patient was homeless or had no family, we had to call on a social worker to help us obtain information about the patient. If a patient could not talk or walk, or simply had an education level below fourth grade, we spent much time gathering information to optimally treat the patient. This scenario was usually the case. We used dry-erase boards, for example, and had the patients write down all their complaints and questions. This process took an extended amount of time.

At 10:30 a.m., all medical residents met for one hour to discuss an interesting case we encountered that day, such as Wegener's granulomatosis, a rare condition that can cause kidney, sinus, and lung problems. One resident presented the case and the other residents contributed to the discussion to help determine the diagnosis. The chief resident (a resident who took an extra year to teach and be a leader among his fellow residents) led the discussion and asked the residents questions throughout this hour, so there never really was a time to relax. We could eat our lunch at this time, as long as nurses, patients, or family members did not need our help.

At 11:30 a.m., we returned to the floor to order radiology studies, draw blood that techs were unable to draw, think about patients' care, review follow-up tests we ordered, and formulate a plan to continue to treat the patients or discharge them from the hospital. This part of the day also involved keeping family members informed, answering pages from nurses about patient care, and responding to other patients in the hospital who required emergency care.

At noon each day, there was another conference where experts talked about a specific condition. Unfortunately, given our workload, we often missed this conference, but tried to attend as many as we could, as they were great opportunities to learn more. Unfortunately, the burdens of sick patients and the need to discharge them or attend to their needs surpassed the desire to sit down for an hour and listen to the lecture. And remember, we are not making easy decisions. We are synthesizing all the information we learned from our four years of medical school to make life and death decisions in addition to the little stuff.

It was now 5:00 p.m., which meant I would be admitting new patients to the hospital from the ER—an average of 5 patients per doctor per call. Other resident physicians would sign out to me to take care of their patients overnight, providing a written synopsis of each patient and how to best care for that patient if an acute issue were to arise. On average, I covered 40 patients and admitted new patients from 5:00 p.m. until 6:00 a.m. the next morning. This meant responding to approximately 10 pages per hour involving patient care in addition to seeing new sick patients. These pages included everything from asking for a diet order to calling about a patient who could not breathe or was dying. I did not rest at all during the first night of call. I remember typing into a computer at 3:00 a.m. with my co-intern John two seats over. We could not believe how much work we had done already, and how much more we had to do.

We kept plugging away and with due diligence, finished our five admissions. Then, since we had not eaten in hours, we scrambled down to the cafeteria to buy a Wendy's sandwich. At 6:00 a.m., my colleagues returned to resume the care of their patients. I gave them the sign out from the previous night, then pre-rounded on the new patients I admitted as well as patients I had been caring for. I was now on hours 24–26 without any sleep. Then, just as the previous day, I rounded with the attending doctor from 8:00 a.m. until 10:30 a.m. At 10:30 a.m., I attended morning report for an hour, and then got back to work, discharging patients, following up on lab results and CT scans, confirming that certain studies were ordered, and answering pages from nurses. I finally got to head home at about 5:00 p.m.

During my 33-hour call night, I did not sleep. After about 24 hours straight of being busy with patients, I began to feel light-headed and my concentration declined a bit, but given the number of patients who needed help and the opportunities for learning, I couldn't afford to sleep. Patients get sick at all hours of the day, not just from 8:00 a.m. to 5:00 p.m. There were times when I wished I had more time to work. We became conditioned to work under all kinds of adverse conditions, despite hunger and lack of sleep. This made us stronger; it gave us the thick skin and the work ethic we needed to accomplish anything. And it paid off in the future, as everything beyond residency seemed easy compared to the rigors we endured during those fateful three years. What's more, my colleagues and I became great friends, fellow warriors with whom I went into battle every day to care for our nation's sick.

Notable Events

After completing my first call cycle, time seemed to fly by. Because I was on call every fourth night for 10 months of my year-long internship, I often did not know what month it was, let alone what day. I still remember wanting more hours in the day just so I could finish the enormous amount of work that needed to be done. The reason this work was magnified deals with the unpredictability of human lives. Patients can get very ill at any time of the day and we need to be there to respond and help them. I remember calling Jackie one night to tell her that I would be home in 10 minutes. Four hours later, I walked through the door. A patient had gotten sick or a family arrived at the hospital and I needed to talk with them or a radiologist called me with a significant finding from a CT just as I was getting into my car and I needed to return to the hospital and order the next test. The term "residents" actually means we live there.

When I came home after call nights, I arrived at around 3:00 p.m. and tried to stay up to talk with Jackie and spend time with my new son. Unfortunately, I often fell asleep as soon as I hit the couch. I woke up confused around 7:00 or 8:00 p.m., ate dinner, and then fell back asleep around 10 p.m., before starting it all over again. I really had no idea what was going on in the world outside work; I caught glimpses of the news at home, but that was rare.

Working at the VA

I worked through different one-month blocks during my first year as an intern. Four of those months were general medicine, including two months at the Veterans Administration down the road. Other one-month blocks included hematology, gastroenterology, cardiology, ICU medicine (two months), and pulmonary. A couple of these months deserve some reflection.

My month with the Veterans Administration (VA) was very rewarding. It was an honor to take care of war veterans, and I admired all of my VA patients. These men and women were selfless and rarely complained. They didn't expect much because they were used to surviving on so little. And, they were optimistic, no matter how sick they were. For example, I remember a particular patient who had lung cancer and was admitted with pneumonia. When I saw him every morning, he was reading the paper with a smile on his face. Instead of feeling sorry for himself, he played cards with his roommate.

Having said that, the higher prevalence of smoking, obesity, and mental disorders among some of my veteran patients made this rotation more challenging. For example, in patients who smoke, wounds and common infections don't heal as easily as they might in a nonsmoker. In addition, the resources and the staff in the VA hospital didn't offer as much help as in other hospitals. Consequently, we did a lot more "scut work" there than in other rotations. Scut work is a term that describes work that should not be done by a doctor, but rather by an administrative person or a technician/nurse, such as drawing blood, making beds, and contacting the radiology department about tests. This scut work took time away from our patients, but was just a part of residency. In the end, it forced us to learn how to multitask, which made us stronger. On a positive note, my memories of the VA included enjoying late-night burritos from Los Tios, a local Mexican carry-out restaurant.

Jackie and I welcomed our first son during this busy time. I was post-call at the VA when she went into labor. Running on empty, with no sleep in the previous 30 hours, I drove Jackie to the Children's Hospital one mile down the road. Within a few hours, our son was born, healthy and happy. This was one of the proudest moments of my life. I had three days of paternity leave, which I cherished tremendously.

My Gastroenterology Rotation

Another month worth highlighting was my gastroenterology rotation. My fourth-year medical student rotation had piqued my interest in this specialty of medicine. At the University of Michigan, we had a full rotation devoted to the care of gastrointestinal and liver diseases. Many other programs did not offer this, nor did they have the large faculty that Michigan had. This rotation was difficult because of a rule that forced us to admit more patients than was the norm. Each intern typically admitted 5 new patients. Once we admitted 5 new patients (and followed 12 patients total), we were said to have "capped." That meant we admitted the maximum number of patients for that call cycle and could admit no more.

Well, the gastroenterology/hepatology rotation was a bit different (as were pulmonary and hematology/oncology). We could get what we called "cap busters." If patients who were on the liver transplant list needed to be admitted, we still had to admit them regardless of our cap, making our total admissions 6 or 7 patients instead of the standard 5 patients. These patients could be admitted at any time, which meant if I had to pre-round starting at 6:00 a.m. and got an admission at 4:00 a.m., I had to do the admission and treat my other 12 patients before 6:00 a.m. And of course, I still had to run codes and tend to the other 60 patients I was covering on service—on no sleep. Although this rotation was challenging, I learned a tremendous amount by caring for these sick patients with end-stage liver disease. Excellent attending doctors mentored me on this rotation, which amplified my desire to pursue gastroenterology as a career.

I remember taking care of a patient with cirrhosis of the liver. When a person's liver does not function correctly, all other organ systems are affected as well. Therefore, when they were admitted to the hospital, I had to address every organ system, including the kidneys, heart, and brain. I viewed this as a challenge, but knowing the complex physiology of the human body allowed me to apply what I had learned in medical school to care for these patients.

Unfortunately, many of these patients needed a liver transplant. The liver transplant process also intrigued me, given all the complexities involved, including the patients' social, physical, and mental states. After my gastroenterology rotation, I knew that the combination of figuring out complex liver patients and the technology of performing endoscopies sealed my interest. In addition, the fact that I could help fight cancer with a screening colonoscopy while also keeping a patient-physician relationship with my Crohn's patients gave me the diversity I was looking for. Finally, using endoscopy to treat life-threatening illnesses such as variceal bleeding (patients with liver disease throwing up large amounts of blood) made the field appealing.

CHAPTER 9

My Second Year of Residency— June 2006–June 2007

I SURVIVED MY FIRST YEAR OF RESIDENCY. I made it through the overnight call, 33-hour work days, 100-hour work weeks, not knowing what day it was, not knowing when my next day off would be. I made it through eating granola bars on the elevator and formulating histories on patients at all hours of the night. I made it through the wide spectrum of emotions, from the pain of patients dying, to the relief that patients survived a critical illness. I was able to continue to have a relationship with my wife and newborn son despite a schedule that did not allow me to return home every fourth night.

I survived this necessary evil called internship. I call it necessary because this training was vital to ensuring I became an expert in caring for our nation's sick, that I was able to function at all hours of the day and act rationally and wisely with a human life in my hands. When one is pushed that hard and forced to use their humility, physical stamina, knowledge, and common sense while keeping their raw emotions in check, one becomes a versatile, well-trained individual—a warrior, as my high school coach would say. The second year of residency required us to use the skills we learned in our first year to become leaders on a team. It also trained us to be more autonomous and make even more independent decisions. As residents, we made the calls, the life and death decisions.

I began my second year of training with the general medicine rotation. I was in charge of two interns (first-year residents), each of whom took care of 12 patients. "In charge" means making sure every single point was accounted for on a daily basis. If interns forgot to do something or were overwhelmed or needed instruction, it was the resident's job to help them. This seems like a manageable job, except for a few points that make the job more difficult than it appears to be.

First, interns usually had 24 hours off in a given week. That meant I would need to take care of my two interns' patients two days out of the week, including their scut work, which was time-consuming. I also supervised the other intern on my team and all of his or her patients. That often meant helping with procedures or other tasks so he or she could go home by 2:00 p.m., catch up with the family, and then crash.

In terms of procedures, every resident is required to do a certain number of procedures before graduating residency—for example, a lumbar puncture (sticking a needle into someone's spine to extract spinal fluid), thoracenteses (sticking a needle into the lung cavity to extract fluid), and central lines (inserting a catheter into the large neck veins to allow fluid to be given). All of these require practice and can be life-threatening if not done properly.

Residents often supervise and help the interns with these procedures, as it takes much practice to do them effectively. These procedures usually take 30–45 minutes to perform. In an ideal world, the nurse would set up all the equipment at the patient's bedside, page the intern when ready, and then be there to assist. The resident would then walk in and provide support. In reality, the intern usually had to walk to three different rooms on three different floors to retrieve all the tools for the required procedure. Often, a room did not have the tool needed. Nurses often were in another patient's room and not available. And, just when the intern was ready to start a procedure, some other issue often arose that delayed the process. Sometimes, the patient needed to use the restroom or families wanted to be updated or the supervising resident was doing another urgent procedure in another location.

From the Resident's Perspective

Most interns were so overwhelmed that it was necessary to step in and help out so they could go home eventually. As an illustration, I will run through a typical patient hospital stay from a resident's perspective. The resident is paged from the ER about an admission. Let's use an easy admission such as pneumonia. The resident decides which intern will be admitting the patient. After the resident notifies the intern via a page, the intern walks to the ER and begins to scour the computer records to get a rough history on the patient. Most often, the records are not in the computer, so the intern may have to call another hospital or a doctor's office, or try to get accurate information from the patient about his or her medical condition.

This process usually takes 30 minutes, given the volume of paperwork. (Some patients have more than 500 pages of documents to sift through based on other medical conditions.) This work also depends on the availability of a computer. Computers can be hard to come by, and I often searched for one for as much as five minutes, and when I found one, I crossed my fingers that it worked.

After acquiring as much medical information as possible, the intern walks to the patient's room to ask the patient questions and perform a physical exam. Even this part is not as straightforward as it sounds. Often, the patient is not in his or her room, and instead is getting an x-ray in the radiology department, at the lab getting blood drawn, or already moved to a different room in the hospital eight floors away. Once the intern finds the patient in his or her room, the intern hopes the patient can talk about and understand his or her medical condition. Unfortunately, this rarely is the case. Patients often can't communicate their medical history due to sickness and pain or a lack of insight about their disease. Maybe there's a language barrier. Older patients often are hard of hearing. Other patients or families are demanding and it takes extra effort to elicit an accurate history. There might be no family members with the patient, or there may be several family members present, each with a different take on the situation, which is often counterproductive.

By the time the intern has found the patient, talked to the patient and the family members, with all the roadblocks mentioned, he or she is down another 20–30 minutes. And this does not include pages and calls about the other 11 patients. Then, the intern places the orders for the patients (i.e., order antibiotics, give fluids, order lab tests, order x-rays, and order home medications). Even finding the home medications is challenging, as the computer system often is outdated or the information is inaccurate.

Finally, the intern must type the "history and physical." This is the 3–5-page document that outlines the patient's reason for being at the hospital; the medical, social, and family history; physical exam findings; labs and radiology findings; and finally, the assessment and plan of action for the patient. This process puts them back another 30 minutes, assuming they are fast typists.

All in all, the process of admitting one patient takes about 90 minutes, assuming there are no other urgent calls or interruptions. I just described one patient, yet an intern had to take care of 12. One can see how an intern can get overwhelmed and why the resident doctor had to assist and mentor the intern.

The discharge process is equally complex. All the stars have to align for it to go smoothly. The social workers have to make sure the health insurance companies and family members are aware the patient is being discharged. All the patient's medications and supplies must be organized and approved by the patient's insurance. A determination must be made about whether the patient is stable enough to leave the hospital. And finally, discharge requires completion of a large document that summarizes the course of the patient's illness from admission to discharge. This document is typically 5–10 pages, depending on the length of the hospital course.

All of these tasks, especially the medications and supplies checklist, are very laborious. Often times, residents have to make several calls to pharmacies and talk with the patient about how to take these medications. Therefore, the resident doctor has to assist in some of these tasks, especially dealing with other demands from other patients, following up on radiology results, or helping to discharge a patient. This "supervising" is stressful because it is the resident's role to make sure the interns get out of work on time, especially since they are working 80–100 hours per week.

In addition to supervising the interns and often doing much of their work, residents were in charge of educating them. This involved bringing in articles about new treatments and challenging them about their patients. For example, if an intern thought a patient was short of breath due to a heart problem, the resident would ask esoteric questions about 30 other causes of shortness of breath. And if the intern didn't know them, the resident would educate him or her in the minutes they had in between taking care of the patients. Other residents' tasks included "running codes." This meant that when a code was called (an alarm that signals that a patient has lost consciousness and/or stopped breathing/heart stopped), the resident was the first one there and called all the shots. In a hospital setting, this happened at least once per call night. It involved sprinting to the room, gathering information about the patient, starting CPR, and then administering orders. This obviously had to be done expeditiously in order to save the patient's life. Several other hospital workers were on the scene, including other doctors, nurses, social workers, and people recording events during the code.

Unfortunately, more often than not, after aggressively trying your hardest for 30 minutes, the code was called and the patient was pronounced dead. Families had to be informed and death paperwork filled out. In the middle of all of this, of course, new pages were coming in about new patients to admit to the hospital. This process takes a physical and emotional toll, as you must control your emotions minutes after filling out death paperwork so you can admit another sick patient. It takes much emotional stamina to deal with death and dying on a nightly basis while trying to explain to families the reasons for illness and death.

The one good thing about this is that time flies by. As I mentioned, a resident doctor actually wishes that time would slow down so he or she would have enough time to finish all the work for that night and to be at rounds the next morning at 7:00 a.m. This is in contrast to other fields where people look at the clock hoping time will fly by so they could go home.

Doing Research

Just when we thought we had no other responsibilities, we had another one. Out of our class of 35, most had aspirations to become specialists. This meant that after our three years of residency, we had to enroll in another two- to three-year fellowship program to learn a specific field of internal medicine, such as gastroenterology or cardiology. Because admissions to fellowships in these specialist fields are competitive, we had to find ways to distinguish ourselves from other excellent candidates. One way to do that was by doing research to demonstrate your competence, work ethic, and commitment to go above and beyond the normal work of a resident.

During our intern year and the first half of our second year, we somehow had to make the time to find a mentor and perform research. This involved brainstorming a question to answer about an area of medical interest, performing a literature search on the current articles available, formulating a clinical question to explore, performing the research, and ultimately writing the paper.

Because my interest was in gastroenterology, and probiotics were a hot topic at the time, I chose to perform a systematic scientific review of all the available probiotics and their efficacy. This meant spending about 20 hours per week reviewing the available literature using our medical databases of the thousands of current studies on probiotics. I spent more hours narrowing my search to approximately 40 studies that were considered quality studies based on certain criteria. I met with my mentors weekly (usually at night), and began analyzing each study and writing the 30-page paper to be submitted for publication. I performed this extra research work in between the long hours in the hospital and taking call. So not only was I working 100 hours per week, I also spent about 10–20 hours per week performing my research.

Fellowship Interview Process
January 2006—March 2006

Most residents choose to move on to a specialty fellowship after completing the internal medicine residency. During the second half of our second year of residency, we began to interview for some of these fellowships. We had just finished the most physically and emotionally demanding year of our lives as interns. Now, just a year later, we were immersed in complete chaos in terms of balancing work, travel, and a home life. We worked hard to build up our resumes (we call it our curriculum vitae, or CV). Now, we had to apply to several fellowship programs, get invited for an interview, and then find a way to travel to—and pay for—the interviews. This was not easy physically, mentally, financially, or emotionally. Let me describe the process.

During our second year of residency, while performing all the tasks mentioned earlier, we had to fill out up to 40 applications to different fellowships throughout the country. Because gastroenterology is competitive and most programs only take between two and four fellows, we had to apply broadly. In 2006, much of this process involved electronic applications; however, each fellowship required a supplemental application, three letters of recommendation, and description of one's research. So in between our overnight calls and patient follow up, we had to find time to talk with our mentors and complete all of these applications. And, we had to find a way to pay for this. We were making about $37,000/year and most of us were supporting families on top of the heavy workload and large student loan burden (mine at $196,000). Each application was approximately $60, so that totalled $2,400 for me—plus the cost of the flight or gas for the car ride.

In January, we began to receive invitations for interviews. I chose to interview at 18 of my top choices, given the competitive nature of gastro-enterology at the time. That meant juggling 18 car rides or flights with long work weeks and no sleep in order to do these interviews. I remember one interview vividly. I had to travel to Wake Forest in North Carolina one day in March. I was going to be post-call the day before the interview and got someone to cover me the following day. My friend and colleague had the same interview day, which meant we were going to work 24 hours the day before the interview, get off work by noon the next day, and drive to North Carolina. Somehow we were able to pull this off by taking turns driving for more than 600 miles.

The interviews for fellowships were relatively predictable. They began with an introduction from the program director about the fellowship. Next, each interviewee (usually about 20 candidates from across the country) broke off and interviewed with different staff at the respective institution. Because gastroenterology is a small world, the conversations usually started off with a question about our mentors and our relationship with them, and the research we were working on. Next, we usually talked about family and the reason we thought their institution was attractive and why it matched our goals. We would meet with about three faculty members, and then have lunch. After lunch, there was usually a tour and the day would be over. Then, in this particular case, we drove 600 miles home to be ready for work the following day.

Looking back, that was crazy, but it was what we had to do. We were doctors and had to make it work. So I ended up going on all of these interviews throughout the second half of my second year of residency. Most often, I drove because it was cheaper. Remember, the money to cover these interviews was coming out of our pockets from our meager salary as residents. I also used my vacation days for interviews. I took two weeks off later that March and went on eight interviews over two weeks.

After spending about $5,000 that we didn't have on interview travel and fees, I ranked my fellowships. I ranked Michigan locations higher, since my extended family was rooted in the metro Detroit area. Fellowships in Michigan included Henry Ford Hospital, Providence Hospital, and William Beaumont Hospital.

When I went on my Henry Ford interview, I felt like it just clicked. I met the program director early that morning and had very down-to-earth conversations. The program was clinically oriented versus research oriented. I really enjoyed taking care of patients, so I wanted a program that would expose me to a variety of pathology and give me experience doing advanced procedures. I did enjoy research, but the primary reason I chose to become a doctor was to help others and watch their progress. Henry Ford was located in downtown Detroit, so a lot of the inner city pathology was encountered there. This created ideal learning opportunities for fellows because we saw the worst consequences of diseases. After the interview, I believed this was the place for me.

Fast forward to June of our second year, and Match Day #2! We had matched for residency programs three years prior, and now it was time to do it again. It was not as dramatic this time, as not all specialties matched on the same day and not all residents chose to specialize. I remember sitting at home on my laptop on my deck when I got the news that I matched at Henry Ford Hospital. I was elated, as I knew I would receive a great clinical experience.

CHAPTER 10

My Third Year of Residency— June 2007–June 2008

Y THIRD AND FINAL YEAR OF RESIDENCY focused more on electives to hone our skills in the area we intended to pursue. Electives are month-long rotations that each resident can "elect" to do. I enjoyed gastroenterology and had just matched, so I chose to do extra months on the gastroenterology consult service to get exposed to a greater variety of patients and better prepare for my profession. I also took a month elective in nephrology (kidney disease) because I always found this field interesting. In addition to these electives, we did our general medicine months, serving as senior residents.

My third year of residency allowed even more autonomy. I spent many months at the VA hospital, where we basically functioned as attending physicians. Attending physicians are the staff doctors who have completed all their respective training and are ultimately in charge of the patients on a team. My attending for the general medicine month at the VA was a previous co-resident who had graduated the year prior to me and chose to stay on as faculty at the VA. I had so much autonomy during that rotation that she simply "ran the list" with me once in the morning and that was it. We sat down and talked about each patient on our list of about 15–20 patients whom I was managing with the help of two interns.

My goal as a senior third-year resident was to teach the interns and make sure everything was getting done in a timely, high-quality manner. At this point in my career, I believed that all those long nights and the quality of training I received at the University of Michigan came together. I had become a chiseled, well-intentioned doctor with the ability to effectively manage a multitude of patients. I really believed I could manage almost everything that was presented to me; nothing surprised me.

For example, as third-year residents, we were in complete charge of codes. Because we had been trained so well and so often with these codes, I no longer got excited when I heard the intercom blast "Code blue. Room 438. Code blue. Room 438." I was able to quickly and calmly assess the situation and manage the patient in a way that gave him or her the best chance of survival. It is truly amazing how humans can get used to anything. I went from worrying about having my lunch money in grade school to worrying about how to save another human life while 10 people were scampering about trying to get all the information and equipment necessary to bring someone back to life in a matter of seconds or minutes. Even though the outcomes for these codes are dismal, chance does favor the prepared mind. As quoted in my favorite book, *The House of God*, "During a code, take your own pulse first."

We also took on a large teaching role during our third year. During our VA rotation, we led morning report. This was the 10:00 a.m. meeting with the residents, fellows, and an attending physician. The interns usually presented interesting cases that they admitted the night before. The senior resident knew about the case before the report and had pertinent medical literature to lead the discussion. We discussed the differential diagnoses (other causes for similar symptoms) and treatment plans for the cases that the interns presented.

It was also a time to talk about "zebras." Zebras are rare diagnoses that medical students read about and get tested on in medical school, but rarely see in actual practice. For example, patients who have shortness of breath often have trouble with their heart or lungs. However, there are other rare conditions that can cause shortness of breath with no issues related to the heart and lungs. At our morning reports, this was the time to bring those up and discuss all possibilities in detail. It was an excellent exercise because it kept our knowledge base current and allowed us to think outside the box.

Research was another important aspect of our third year of residency. We had been working hard since our intern year trying to develop research. Now was the time to display our research projects to the whole program. We prepared posters of our projects during April of our last year of residency, working on them in between our calls and all our other patient care responsibilities. My research project focused on different probiotics and their impact on a common condition called irritable bowel syndrome.

A co-fellow and I began this project my intern year by browsing thousands of articles from a complex search engine medical professionals use. After spending months analyzing these articles and determining which ones were high quality, we narrowed them down to about 30. Determining which ones were quality is a whole course and career itself. Suffice it to say, it involved daily rigorous analysis with occasional meetings with our mentor. These meetings were notoriously difficult to secure. We typically had to meet with him during inconvenient times, such as 7:00 p.m. My co-fellow and I would knock on his door at the VA hospital and he would answer, often eating soup straight out of the can or lettuce straight from the bag. We very efficiently went over our work, he gave us some brief words of encouragement, and we carried on.

Carry on. The goal was to take each day at a time, as our journey was so long. And this mentality did pay off. In three years, I went from a timid intern thrown into a sea of uncertainty to a well-trained doctor capable of handling some of the most complex urgent medical issues in a calm, collected manner. If I actually thought about the fact that I had three more years of substandard pay, frequent calls, and larger debt burden, I would have driven myself crazy.

CHAPTER 11

My First Year of Gastroenterology Fellowship— June 2008–July 2009

A FEW DAYS AFTER RESIDENCY ENDED, I moved on to my fellowship. My family and I relocated from Ann Arbor to the Metro Detroit area so I would be closer to Henry Ford Hospital. This was our third move in seven years. We found a modest ranch home about 25 miles from Henry Ford so my wife could still be close to Ann Arbor, where she was teaching at the university. We had bought the condo in Ann Arbor in 2005. Unfortunately, it was now 2008 and the recession hit home prices hard. To avoid losing $30,000, which we could not afford, we decided to rent our condo out via an ad on Craigslist. Luckily, we were able to rent it out to an incoming resident, but prior to his arrival, I had to do some work on the condo, such as painting the deck, doing a thorough cleaning, and making simple repairs—all in the midst of moving my family 30 miles east.

Fellowship started on July 1, 2008—one day after residency ended. It was time to learn new computer systems, get acquainted with a new large hospital, and meet my co-fellows. Fellowship is much different than residency. First, the class sizes are smaller. I had three other fellows in my class and there were three classes total. (Our residency class had about 35 residents in each class.) Second, in fellowship, we focus mainly on our chosen specialty, which was gastroenterology and hepatology. This field studies the internal organs, including the esophagus, stomach, small and large intestines, liver, pancreas, and gallbladder. The field requires three extra years of training because we not only learn about these organs in great detail, we need to become experts in performing endoscopy. Endoscopy includes colonoscopies, upper endoscopies, and many other specialized advanced procedures. During this fellowship, we completed more than 2,000 procedures in addition to taking care of our patients in the clinic and in the hospital and performing research.

I remember my first day well. The nurse coordinator taught us about performing upper endoscopy, which involves advancing a long thin scope about the diameter of one pinky finger into the mouth of a patient. The scope is maneuvered into the esophagus, then into the stomach, then all the way to the first portion of the small intestine. The goal is to examine the small intestine, stomach, and esophagus. The procedure is commonly used to diagnosis reflux disease, stomach ulcers, and cancers, or to take samples for conditions such as celiac disease.

The description seems relatively straightforward, but the intricacy of the instrument actually made it daunting. Adding to that a live breathing person that we are sedating, it becomes a rather complex procedure. We started off the first few days by practicing with video simulators to get an idea of how to use the dials to maneuver the scope. It takes about 100 experiences to feel like one is getting the hang of it. It takes a full three years of performing these procedures daily to become an expert.

On my second day, I saw patients in the hospital and treated their gastrointestinal ailments. In contrast to residency, where I often called a consult to get a specialist to perform a given procedure, I was the one being consulted by the hospital services. Our consult team included me and a senior fellow. Our team was managed by our attending doctor, who assisted us when procedures got difficult or when we had questions regarding consults. He also heard our presentations and agreed or disagreed with our assessments.

Consult blocks were broken up into months, similar to residency. I did eight months on the GI consult team, and three months on hepatology the first year, with one month off. On a typical day on the consult service I arrived at 6:30 a.m. to follow up on the patients we were following—about 15 overall. I stopped by each room, performed a physical exam, and decided on the plan. Meanwhile, beginning at 8:00 a.m., we started to get new consults—typically between 6 and 12 per day. They came in for complaints such as blood in the stool, abdominal pain, pancreatitis, and trouble swallowing.

When I received the electronic page, I called the doctor to find out why I was needed for the consult. I then went to see the patient. I walked through the maze of the hospital in search of the patient's room. When I arrived, I interviewed the patient, performed a physical exam, did a rectal exam to assess the severity of bleeding (in the case of blood in the stool, for example), and decided whether we needed to perform an endoscopy. This assessment took about 30 minutes.

After I talked to my attending and if he agreed to perform the endoscopy, I notified our nurses so they could call the patient to our endoscopy area. Once the patient was in the area and was ready, we wheeled the patient into the room, consented him or her, and performed the procedure. This whole process took another 45 minutes. Of course, during the process, we got innumerable pages about other new consults or from patients we had already seen.

Just like residency, nothing was easy. Often, the consent was difficult to obtain because the patient was so sick he or she couldn't talk, or didn't speak English, or had dementia. In these cases, we had to call the guardian or interpreter services, which added precious time to each case. Again, learning to multitask in residency paid dividends here. Even worse, when we were performing the procedures, we could not simply stop and check the pager. Often times, we would come back to three or four pages that we had to respond to right after the procedure. Only then could we do the procedure report, call the doctor who called the consult, and see other new consults. This process went on throughout the day. Each day became easier and easier as we got more accustomed to the procedures.

Our first 50 upper endoscopies were humbling. We went from being confident about managing any urgent patient medical condition in residency to barely being able to hold the scope properly in fellowship. Patience and persistence were important traits to have during this trying time. The experience of hearing your pager going off, trying to learn a brand new procedure while keeping your sedated patient safe, and having the answer to the patient's problem proved difficult. As specialists, we had to have the answer—there was no one else to go to after us. Some attending doctors allowed us to spend time trying to figure out how to maneuver the scope; others were less patient. We just had to adapt and learn from the previous experience.

In addition to our daily work, we took call every eighth night from 5:00 p.m. until 7:00 a.m. In contrast to residency, we actually went home during that time and came in only if there was an urgent call, such as patients getting food stuck in their esophagus, patients vomiting blood, or patients having severe liver failure. However, just like residency, we had to work the day leading up to call and the next day as well.

For example, on my call day, I worked from 6:30 a.m. until 5:30 p.m., and then started taking call until 7:00 a.m. the next day. This made for a very long day. And if I had to go into the hospital at 2:00 a.m., I still had to be back at the hospital at 6:30 a.m. the following day. You can imagine how difficult it was if we did get called in at night. This happened about half the time. During call, in addition to getting urgent pages, we received calls from patients who had questions. Anything could come our way and we had to be prepared. We did not sleep well, often awakened by the harsh noise of our pager. It was a time when dinner was interrupted to answer a page or I was unable to attend my kids' sporting events. The pager could go off at any moment, ultimately sending me back to the hospital at 2:00 a.m.

During my second month, I was on the liver (hepatology) service, where I saw some of the sickest patients in the hospital. These patients often had advanced liver disease due to alcohol, hepatitis C, or fatty liver. Unfortunately, there is no magic pill or cure once a patient develops scarring or cirrhosis of the liver. They often are admitted to the hospital due to complications from the disease, such as confusion related to liver toxins, vomiting blood from esophageal varices, or an infection. In addition, Henry Ford is a liver transplant center; they performed about 100 liver transplants each year when I was a fellow there. With that came responsibilities to manage these patients after the transplant as well. They were on multiple medications and the patients often ran into problems after the transplant, such as rejection of the liver they received.

A typical day on the hepatology service was as follows: I arrived at the hospital at 5:30 a.m. with my senior fellow. We averaged about 25 patients on our list and about eight new consults per day. We usually split this workload evenly. At 5:30 a.m., we began pre-rounding. This three- to four-hour process involved evaluating each patient before we met with our attending doctor for actual rounds. When I arrived at the hospital, I logged onto the computer and printed all the labs and new radiology studies that patients received the previous night, which amounted to about five sheets of information per patient. I then went to each patient's room, one by one. I asked them how the night was and if anything urgent occurred. I performed a full physical exam. After the exam, I asked the nurse how the night went for that patient. I recorded the vital signs and other important parameters. I gathered all my labs, the nurse's notes, and my history and physical exam, and wrote out a SOAP note—a one-page assessment of the patient's current condition, including our recommendations for the day.

On a good day, each patient took about 20 minutes to pre-round on. Most times, however, the correct labs were not drawn. Or the vital signs or other parameters were not recorded. Or the patient's paper chart could not be found. Or the patient was off the floor. Or I received a page about some other patient or a new consult. Or new family members were at the patient's bedside and needed an update. So many factors had to be prioritized during the process of seeing patients in the morning. Residency trained us to be efficient and I am thankful for that.

After about four hours of diligently evaluating these patients as well as the new consults for the day, we returned to our division floor to meet with our attending doctor and accompany him or her on rounds. For each patient, we presented our findings from our pre-rounding by using our SOAP note as a reference. During rounds, we received calls about transfers of patients from other hospitals or new consults throughout the day. At 11:00 a.m., we met with the surgeons to discuss plans for patients who had already undergone a liver transplant. At noon, we picked up where we left off and continued rounding throughout the day. Sometimes, we performed an upper endoscopy for bleeding or pain.

At 4:30 p.m., we all gathered in a lecture hall to hear about an exciting topic on our field. These topics were researched and presented by the fellows. Yes, in addition to our busy call nights and days, we were responsible for producing an hour-long lecture using PowerPoint about four times per year on various topics related to our field. My topic during my first year was Wilson's disease, a rare liver disorder that results in abnormal deposition of copper in the liver. I spent at least 15 hours researching the disease. I did this research at night, when I got home from a long day of rounding. The staff physicians often asked us questions about our topic and we had to be prepared to answer them based on our research. It was a good experience because in addition to teaching us how to conduct efficient research, it prepared us for public speaking.

Because I was so busy my first year of fellowship, it flew by. Soon enough, I was entering my second of three years of fellowship.

CHAPTER 12

My Second Year of Fellowship— June 2009– July 2010

O UR SECOND YEAR OF FELLOWSHIP was similar to the first. We got more exposure to the consult services and took on more of a supervisory role, being in charge of the first-year fellows on the consult teams. During our second year, we also were trained in colonoscopy, which is technically more difficult than upper endoscopy.

The colon appears in diagrams as a straight tube. In reality, it is a very twisty tubular structure. This procedure mainly is done to screen for colon cancer and to remove colon polyps. However, it is also used to diagnose causes of gastrointestinal bleeding, diarrhea, or abdominal pain.

During our consult months, we did all the colonoscopies with the supervision of our attending doctors. The goal is to insert the colonoscope all the way from the rectum to the end of the colon where it connects with the small intestine. Getting to the end is the part that requires about 1,000 colonoscopies to be considered well-trained. During our first 100 colonoscopies, it took about 30 minutes to get to the end, with many errors made along the way. By the end of our training, we could routinely get to the end in about 5 minutes.

This complex procedure requires dexterity of the hands and a vision to maneuver the colon without causing pain. Safety is another issue in relation to this procedure. If not done correctly, there is a risk of tearing (perforating) the bowel wall. Learning this procedure was analogous to stepping into the hospital on my first day of residency: like a deer in headlights. Only with persistence and patience was I able to accomplish my goals in training.

In addition to presenting lectures for our division, maintaining the consult services, and doing overnight calls, we were required to participate in research. I was even more heavily involved in fellowship research, as I was interested in how the treatment of hepatitis C after patients received a liver transplant would help them. I spent over an hour every day working on this issue from the middle of my first year until about September of my second year of fellowship. I submitted my work and was ecstatic when I was selected to do an oral presentation at an international meeting in Boston in October.

The amount of work to get this presentation just right was daunting. I spent about 100 hours working with a statistician, my mentor, and my laptop to get the presentation the way I wanted it. And of course, this was usually at 10:00 p.m., after we put our kids to bed and I finished a long day at work—which brings up the one benefit of call. Because I was paged so often, I rarely got more than one hour of sleep at a time. So I used that time to work on research. I was never completely satisfied with the presentation, and tweaked it innumerable times. When I did present my research to over 1,000 people from all over the world, I felt very comfortable and nailed it because I had practiced this 20-minute talk so many times. That day, I truly felt that I contributed something extra to the medical field.

Moonlighting

Despite the rigors of being a physician in training, we all tried to have a life outside of medicine. Unfortunately, the years of training took their toll physically, mentally, and financially. We had two children and were expecting a third son in February. During the past couple years, my student loan debt had continued to balloon and despite living a very frugal lifestyle, we had trouble making ends meet.

Luckily, in fellowship, moonlighting opportunities came to light. Moonlighting was an opportunity to make extra money by doing night shifts at the hospital. I would actually be doing hospitalist work in internal medicine—the field I was trained in at the University of Michigan. Initially, this seemed crazy, given so many other tasks involved in fellowship, including overnight call. However, to support my family during this financially trying time, I filled out the hundreds of pieces of paperwork required for this opportunity.

I worked evenings, typically a 6:00 p.m. to 11:00 p.m. shift at the same hospital I was working at. I then worked the next morning for fellowship not related to the moonlighting. I was the one person in my fellowship to do this, as our fellowship itself was very demanding and required at least 70 hours of work per week. Add on another 15 hours per week of moonlighting and you have one full week. But that was nothing that I was not used to. I worked

36-hour shifts and did not come home every fourth night in residency. Everything is relative. The body can do amazing things. I walked out of the hospital at 11:30 p.m. knowing that I would return in about six hours. This was tough, but it helped pay the bills.

There was one moonlighting opportunity I will never forget. I had a week-long vacation coming up in May of my second year. We usually didn't go anywhere on vacations because we could not afford it, but I thought that taking the time off may give me a chance to relax. When I realized night shifts were available at another Henry Ford Hospital in the area, however, my personality and need for extra money took over. The shift was from 7:00 p.m. to 7:00 a.m. for six straight nights. So, sure enough, I spent the entire week of my vacation working over 65 hours. It was something I was wired for and something I thought was right for my family. I have to thank my wife throughout these times, as she was taking care of our kids and working part time at the University of Michigan. We were a great team that always persisted and we still hold that close to our hearts.

CHAPTER 13

My Third Year of Fellowship— June 2010–July 2011

IN JULY 2010, I BEGAN MY THIRD and final year of fellowship. This year was focused on honing all the skills we learned during our first two years. It was also time to start looking for my first real job. That sounded amazing. For the first time since I mowed lawns in college, I was free to look for a regular job and to use my medical schooling and training. This process was daunting and demanded a lot of time.

I used several websites and called gastroenterology groups in the area in the hopes of landing a good job. I started in July 2010 by calling several groups in Michigan and other states to get a good idea of the landscape. This was called "cold calling." I looked up the group online, read the biographies of the partners, and made a decision about calling them. If I called, I typically talked to the gastroenterology group's practice manager. I then emailed my CV to the group. A few days later, one of the members of the gastroenterology practice would call me and talk about common goals, interests, talents, etc. They would gauge my personality and decide whether to offer me a formal interview with the group. This phone conversation usually lasted about an hour.

If mutually agreed upon, I flew or drove to the respective group for the interview. On the day of the interview, I met all the partners at breakfast, lunch, or dinner. In between those times, the practice manager took me to the endoscopy center and to the hospital for a tour. In the evening, we had dinner with all the partners and got to know them—their families work-life balance, etcetera. Sometimes, I went on a second interview if I really enjoyed the place. Eventually, if the group thought I was a great fit, they sent me a contract with the salary and terms of the employment.

During my third year of fellowship, I went on about 12 interviews. I talked to probably 20 groups over the phone and decided they were not a good fit—whether it was based on the location, the group dynamic, their practice patterns, or whether they were ready to take on a new doctor. Again, just like residency, these interviews were on our own time and dime. At this stage, however, some groups did pay for the flight and hotel, which was a big change from residency and fellowship interviews. I often tried to interview on a Friday or Monday so I could drive or fly into the interview and have a weekend day as a travel day and not miss work. If that did not work out, I used the few vacation days I had.

During our years of training, we were never taught about the "business" of medicine. We were busy making sure our patients came first; the outside real world was just a fantasy land where people worked 8:00 a.m. to 5:00 p.m. and had weekends off. Medical school was a microcosmic society of living in the library, only to exit into the real world for lunch or dinner. Aside from a 30-minute lecture about loan consolidation by a financial advisor during our fourth year of medical school, we never had the chance to learn about real-world issues such as loan repayment, investments, and mortgages. We would learn all about it on our own someday—and boy did we.

I interviewed at two types of practices: the employed model and the private practice model. In the employed model, the doctors work for a hospital system and therefore a large multi-specialty medical group. Internal medicine doctors, pulmonologists, hematologists, and surgeons all work as one big team and all share the costs and the revenue. Henry Ford Health System, where I did my fellowship, is such a model. In the private practice model or single-specialty group, the doctors work for themselves or for the private group. The type of practice may include anywhere from one (solo practice) to 20 doctors in the group (single-specialty group). The difference is that all of these doctors are gastroenterologists. They do their own billing, own the endoscopy centers where they perform their procedures, and do not rely on other specialties to bring in revenue. They hire their own nurses and staff.

A negative aspect of a private group practice is that doctors typically must take out a large loan in the hundreds of thousands of dollars in order to buy into the group. Also, they must build up a practice and get primary care doctors to refer their patients to the group.

In general, the benefits of an employed model include not having to "buy into" the group, and arriving on day one with a built-in volume of patients and an automatic referral base of patients. This often means a higher starting salary and a quicker route to higher compensation because of the automatic referral base.

One of the negative aspects of the employed model is that the doctors cannot take ownership into the endoscopy centers, which can generate significant revenue after the loan is paid off. Also, in the employed model, administrators who are not doctors tell doctors how to practice. These administrators also get a slice of the revenue the doctors bring in, even though they never went to medical school. In addition, the doctor-patient relationship is less under the doctor's control in the employed model because the nurses and managers work for the system, not for the doctors. The system, not the doctor, hires the staff. Therefore, if one has a good idea on how to improve access to patients or make things more efficient, it must go through a bunch of red tape.

During my private practice interviews, we talked about how compensation structure worked, how medical insurers paid the group, what other investment opportunities the group had, such as buy ins to the endoscopy center or buildings. In return, assuming I made it as a partner, I would receive some revenue from that endoscopy center to supplement my salary after my loan paid off the buy-in amount. During the employed model interviews, we talked about how the system was doing financially and how the doctor would fit into the larger system.

As you can imagine, I had to do my own research on the "business" of medicine before I started this interview process. After putting the kids to bed at night, I spent countless hours on the Internet learning about buy-in structure, loan types, practice styles, and how insurers actually paid doctors. I found it quite enjoyable because this was my future; this was the culmination of what I had dreamed of as a boy. It was about to become a reality.

After interviewing all over the country, staying in hotels, and taking red eye flights home just in time to work the next day, I decided to stay at Henry Ford. I chose this opportunity because I enjoyed my fellowship tremendously, made some great friends, and learned from some down-to-earth mentors. I also had the opportunity to get additional training in ERCP, which is a scope test procedure that allows us to treat bile duct disorders in the liver. And, Henry Ford was close to my family.

Soon enough, my fellowship was coming to an end. I had done more than 2,000 procedures and saw thousands of consults in preparation to go out on my own. I had taken my last page on call and it was nice to finally retire that pager. This was actually a big deal. That pager had been attached to my belt for six straight years—with the same ringtone throughout. Hearing that ringtone at all hours of the day and night, thousands of times over those six years of training, definitely had an impact on me.

Now, when I hear that ringtone go off from another pager, my heart skips a beat and I get a little nervous because I knew that was me on the front lines not long ago. It was me getting up out of bed to go in and save a life. It was me talking to a sick patient on the phone at 3:00 a.m. about the abdominal pain she'd had for years. It was me waking up, calling back another doctor hundreds of miles away, and helping him manage a sick liver patient. It was me who now had post-traumatic stress from hearing that familiar, startling noise. I still have a pager as a staff gastroenterologist, but it is a different feel. I still get many 2:00 a.m. calls, but the pages are not as frequent. And I definitely changed the ringtone.

CHAPTER 14

Life as a Gastroenterologist— July 2011 to Now

I PASSED THE BOARD EXAM IN NOVEMBER 2011 to become a gastroen-terologist. This $2,500 gastroenterology board exam is yet another test in our quest to become a "real doctor." This is the last exam I have to take until I re-certify in internal medicine in 7 years. I re-certify in gastroenterol-ogy every 10 years. Of course, there are other mandatory medical education courses I must take yearly and conferences I must attend (and money I must spend) in order to keep up with the requirements of board certification.

I now see patients in the office two days a week and I perform procedures three days a week. I take weekend call and weeknight call on a rotating basis. Weekend call is rigorous—similar to fellowship. The positive aspects are that we can make our own decisions and do not have to run everything by an attending doctor. I am enjoying my life and am proud to have made it through this long, arduous journey. I feel like I have met my calling and am serving the greater good. I truly enjoy serving my patients and using my knowledge to help them.

Stresses of the Profession

However, even after training, there are still issues that plague our profession and break us down. These are issues that threaten the hearts of practicing doctors because they add undue stress in an already chaotic environment.

Inconsistent Schedules

One issue involves our lack of a consistent schedule and its effect on our per-sonal lives. Our families never know if we will be home for dinner or whether we can take the kids to soccer practice, which can create stress. It's simply out of our control most of the time.

For example, I usually perform endoscopic procedures from 8:00 a.m. to 5:00 p.m. three days per week. I perform these procedures on 16 patients per day. One day, I finished my second to last case at 4:45 p.m. We were running a bit behind, as usual, due to the increasing amount of computer work required. My last patient felt it was not important to arrive on time—45 minutes prior to his scheduled procedure—and arrived instead at 5:00 p.m. He needed an interpreter, and his required driver chose to leave the site. By the time the nurses were able to assess the patient, place an IV, and do all the pre-operative history, it was 5:30 p.m. By the time I talked with the patient through the interpreter, sedated the patient, and completed the procedure, it was 5:50 p.m. And of course, the patient's driver was not there, so we had to wait for the driver to arrive. I didn't walk out until 6:30 p.m.—90 minutes late.

Sadly, examples like this are typical. Doctors always need to put patients first, which explains why we miss our kids' sporting events or school plays on a fairly regular basis. We do not clock in and out of work. We call back our patients "after work" and make sure they are safe and cared for, at whatever hour that may be. This idea of always being available hurts our health as well as our relationships with our own families. It is a mental war that we battle daily, knowing that we can be paged at any moment. But we are doctors; we can handle it.

Multitasking

Another issue involves the need to multitask constantly. When patients call their doctors, their doctors are busy taking care of patients. Answering their calls, their questions, adds to the stressful work doctors are already doing. The nurse triages the calls, but we still have to read her computer messages and respond to the patients. Often, we call the patient personally and try to figure out over the phone what the next steps are. Because we are seeing patients every half hour, we are doing this additional work at lunch, after work, or in between patients.

For example, I may be calling a patient about her liver failure after I just diagnosed colon cancer in a patient via a colonoscopy. I once received a call at 2:00 a.m. from a patient who had suffered from abdominal pain for three years. She was angry and said no other doctor treated her for this pain. I had never met this patient, but she wanted me to prescribe narcotic pain medication. Although I empathized with her, late-night calls are meant for urgent issues, not issues that have been present for years. These extra pages we answer at night make us more fatigued, disrupt our sleep patterns, and affect us physically the next day. Nothing is harder than having to drive to the hospital at 2:00 a.m. for an urgent bleeding case, return home at 4:00 a.m., and then have to wake up at 6:30 a.m. to work another 11-hour day.

No Downtime

Another related issue is that we are never off-duty—even when we are on vacation. For example, the weekend before Christmas, I had a very busy service. I finished my weekend on Monday morning with plans of having Christmas off. However, during my Christmas vacation, I spent many hours checking my nurse emails and answering pages from other doctors. If patents' results came in while I was on vacation, I talked to them about their diagnoses. I even went in on Christmas Eve to help a colleague. I have given patients' diagnoses over the phone while on vacation. This is what doctors do for their colleagues and patients every day. We are never off from work. I always pack my laptop so I can check patients' results on a nightly basis and place follow-up calls. I have to ensure I have Internet access at all times, as the electronic medical record stalks us without mercy.

Relating to the idea of "never being off from work," we treat patients at all hours of the day. Whether it is driving in during a snowstorm at 3:00 a.m. or driving in to save someone after they choke on Thanksgiving dinner, we are available. We do not get compensated more for treating patients during weekend, holiday, or nighttime hours. I bring this up because of a real-life example related to this "overtime work."

My air conditioner died on a Sunday a few weeks ago. When I called the HVAC service, they stated they charge a double hourly rate on a Sunday. In addition, they charge more than $100 just to pull into the driveway! Furthermore, I knew they can charge whatever they want to, given the demand in the hot weather. I, of course, declined that quote and lived in the heat for two days.

As doctors, *we* do not get paid more for arriving in the middle of the night or working on Sundays or holidays. We are there for our patients no matter what or when. We see them at all times and will never refuse care. I'm frustrated when I hear that a friend was able to get double the hourly pay for working overtime or friends in the service industry can charge a premium on a weekend. But again, we are doctors; we can handle it.

Thankfully, the challenges of residency taught me to be flexible and to remain calm. This job requires patience, persistence, and a level mind. After all, we are trying to help patients at their most vulnerable moments. We need to rely on our own inner strength, training, and knowledge to synthesize a plan for them, no matter when or why they call us. We have to be on at all times.

Rules and Regulations

As if all this weren't enough, we also must deal with institutional regulations that increase our stress and workload. Patient satisfaction scores are one example. Patients now can rate us according to how they think we did at the office or how satisfied they were. Those scores can affect our compensation. But, it is a very subjective system. While I agree that all doctors need to be respectful, patient satisfaction scores have not been shown to improve patient outcomes. In fact, a major study showed that patients who give higher patient satisfaction scores have a higher chance of death!

Our goal as doctors is to heal patients. If giving a pain medication or prescribing an antibiotic is done just to make a patient happy and improve a satisfaction score, there is something wrong. That antibiotic could cause a fatal reaction. We know the results of these surveys are invalid, as patients often comment about things that are not even related to their health. For example, patients have stated that their coffee was not warm enough in the waiting room. Or that the walls in the office did not match. Or that they didn't like a doctor because he was drinking a Diet Coke.

Doctors should not be compared to employees at a hotel resort or a cruise line. Customers have a different mindset on a cruise than they do when they are sick at a doctor's office. People have no problem paying for a $10 margarita, but they do have trouble paying $25 for an office co-pay if they are miserable and sick. We are treating vulnerable sick patients who do not need "customer service." They need to be healed. Patients need to let us use our years of training to help them get better, not to make them satisfied or happy. Patients need to realize that what makes them happy is not always the best care. The emphasis on patient satisfaction pressures doctors to acquiesce to demands for medications or unnecessary diagnostic tests.

I agree that doctors need to be respectful and professional while visiting patients. But to tie compensation to how patients judge me when they are vulnerable is not right. It is hard for patients to be "satisfied" if they are very sick or have chronic pain symptoms and all of the health problems are not fixed at a 30-minute office visit. It is impossible for a patient to know what went into the years of training or the nuances to their disease process in order to know if we did a "good job" or not. The doctor-patient relationship is sacred and complex. It takes time for this to grow. It is not as quick and easy as refreshing a daiquiri on a cruise ship. We are doctors who have trained for 14 years to heal patients and visit with patients during times when they are vulnerable and, frankly, not happy.

Related to this idea is the reputation that doctors are always "late" and that patients wait in the waiting rooms at least 30 minutes to an hour before their appointment, making them unsatisfied and angry. This is true. Patients often wait beyond their normal appointment time. But there is much more going on there than meets the eye. Medicine is not black and white science. It is the art of healing patients at their most vulnerable moments from an emotional and physical standpoint. This art takes time, and some patients take longer than others. An elderly patient who takes 25 medications and needs help using the restroom during the visit takes longer than a 25-year-old with a cold. In our field, 9 out of 10 patients fall into the complex category. One may then wonder why doctors do not account for the time lag. The simple answer to that is that our government wants us to see more patients, do more, document more, get evaluated more, get sued more, yet get compensated less.

M. Dawn Linn, DO, wrote a blog on her Rapha Family Wellness website (www.raphafamilywellness.com/blog) that addresses this issue quite well. It is entitled, "Why in the. . . . does a doctor schedule my appointment for 2:40, and then keep my ass in the office for at least 30 minutes?" Her response to that question:

> While in a perfect world each patient would come in with a simple problem, (i.e., I stubbed my toe, I have poison ivy), they don't. More commonly a day goes like this . . .
>
> Mrs. Jones is 76 and has smoked nearly her entire life. She made an appointment for a lump that she has noticed come up on her arm. A quick visit . . . today. I think they might be nothing but since I'm not sure I send her to a surgeon who also thinks they might be nothing but takes one off anyway. Remember Mrs. Jones because she will come up in a moment.
>
> A few days later I am seeing Mr. Green who is 78 and following up on his thyroid medication. Should be simple enough except

that Mr. Green's wife of 56 years has just passed away. She, too, was my patient. He is crying, unable to sleep, full of anxiety and depressed. I, too, start to cry and console and pray for him right there in the room. Only after we have that discussion are we able to move on to his "medical" care.

One reason we are late: we console.

Right after him I go in to see a chronically uncontrolled diabetic. It would be easy to think that she is simply non-compliant, but the fact is that she cannot afford her medications and so she only takes them every few days. I am aware that there are patient assistance programs available online but she does not have Internet access so I take the time to help her fill out the appropriate paperwork for this.

One reason we are late: we care.

Remember Mrs. Jones? The surgeon is now on the phone and wants to talk to me. Turns out those lumps she had are stage IV lung cancer and he has sent for a CT scan which he is sending the results of to my office. She is at my front desk asking for these results . . . she has no idea she has cancer. So, yes, I work her in, "adding on extra patients at the last minute and it makes everyone suffer." Not only do I get the joy of explaining to her that she has cancer that came up as suddenly as a Spring rain, I get to call her husband on the phone and explain it to him while she cries in my office. I call the oncologist to set up her appointment for the very next day. I get to be the one who tells her that she doesn't have very long to live.

One reason we are late: we take time.

Yes, this was a real day. And, yes, often I am AT LEAST 30 minutes behind, at the very least. That particular day I was 90 minutes behind. But I can guarantee you that not another person that day was upset with me because each of them has learned that I am the type of doctor who would do the exact same thing for each of them.

So the next time your doctor is 30 minutes late, instead of playing Candy Crush or FB on your phone and constantly looking at your clock, look around the office or the waiting room. Say a silent pray for those there with you because you have no idea why they are there, just like they have no clue about what you suffer. But I do. I carry it home with me every night. I work my nurses too hard for too little pay because I demand that my patients are taken care of. They do more than just bring patients back to rooms. They call in your refills, fill out your paperwork, write notes for school or work, find samples and coupons, play with your kids, look up your immunization records, talk to your spouse on the phone who is worried about your recent visit to the ER. Sometimes they spend more than two hours on the phone with an insurance company for Mrs. Little, trying to figure out why they will no longer cover her medication for her multiple sclerosis that has been the only thing that has allowed her to function for the past 5 years. And sometimes I even have to argue about it with somebody on the other line.

One reason we are late: we are advocates.

And, sometimes even the doctor has issues like the day I learned (in the middle of my morning) that my mother had breast cancer. I'm sure you were in the waiting room complaining about my being behind while I was in the bathroom crying and trying to freshen up because I still had patients to take care of.

One reason we are late: we are human.

Yes, in a perfect world, we would never be behind, but we would also ONLY see healthy young people whose biggest complaint is how far behind we are in our schedule. And, while it would be nice to think that your $20 copay is paying for my "bigger McMansion," the truth is that I work 60 hours a week running my own clinic (actually IN the clinic) and another 4 hours every night (after my kids go to bed) and another 12–24 hours in an ER 2 hours away on the weekends in order to pay my staff less than what they deserve and try to chunk away at the $270,000 in student loans that I willingly took on so I could hear people complain about themselves (or me and my office) all day long. Take time to think about that the next time you're waiting 30 minutes and maybe you'll realize that 30 minutes really isn't as long as you think.

Required computer documentation is another example of institutional regulations that hamper our care. Doctors are now consumed with checking boxes, implementing EMRs, and transitioning to a new coding system for billing—all while seeing increasing patient loads and meeting increasingly steep clinical demands. We notice that we now have to document more metrics on the computer that were handed down as a requirement from our institution. Even though we know it doesn't improve health outcomes, we still have to abide by the regulations. This breaks us down for many reasons:

1. Computers freeze intermittently throughout the day. Patients think we are behind, yet we are simply at the mercy of the hour glass on the computer.

2. Increasing documentation requirements pull us away from one-on-one interactions with our patients. It forces us to stare at a screen and document metrics while the patient talks; our patients are not getting better care from this.

3. We have no access to the computer chart during the multiple "down-times" per week. This is poor care, as the medical record is vital to optimal patient care, especially during urgent cases. This hurts that sacred patient-physician relationship. Yet we can handle these setbacks; we are doctors.

CHAPTER 15

Reflections and a Call to Action

MEDICINE IS A UNIQUE PROFESSION FOR MANY REASONS, and I hope I have been able to convey the daunting struggles and challenges doctors face, beginning with that initial decision to enter the field of medicine. With that as a backdrop, I hope the public and our government will consider the effect of policy changes on the doctor's financial well-being.

Let me take you back to my second year of fellowship. I had gone through five years of call, long work hours, mountains of debt, risk of lawsuits, and several moves, all while raising a family. One night on call, when I was feeling a rush of emotions, I wrote down my thoughts and asked a friend of mine to publish it on his blog, Caduceusblog. Fortunately, KevinMD, the largest social media platform for medicine, picked up the blog and published it in March 2013. The article went viral, receiving more than 1 million hits on various websites and 66,000 shares and "likes" on Facebook within four days. It really seemed to hit a nerve with the public. It also had some critics, including lawyers, who thought, "How can he complain when he makes more than most people in the country?"

The article, reprinted below, really summarizes my thoughts.

My Personal Open Letter to Lawmakers:

I am writing this letter because I feel that our leaders and lawmakers do not have an accurate picture of what it actually entails to become a physician today; specifically, the financial, intellectual, social, mental, and physical demands of the profession. This is an opinion that is shared among many of my colleagues. Because of these concerns, I would like to personally relate my own story. My story discusses what it took to mold, educate, and train a young Midwestern boy from modest roots to become an outstanding physician, who is capable of taking care of any medical issues that may plague your own family, friends, or colleagues.

I grew up in the suburbs of southeast Michigan in a middle-class family. My father is an engineer at General Motors and my mother is a Catholic school administrator in my hometown. My family worked hard and sacrificed much to enroll me in a private Catholic elementary school in a small town in Michigan. I thought I wanted to be a doctor in 5th grade based on my love of science and the idea of wanting to help others despite no extended family members involved in medicine. Winning a science fair project about the circulatory system in 6th grade really piqued my interest in the field.

Throughout high school, I took several science courses that again reinforced my interest and enthusiasm toward the field of medicine. I then enrolled at Saint Louis University to advance my training for a total of eight years of intense education, including undergraduate and medical school. The goal was to prepare myself to take care of sick patients and to save the lives of others (four years of undergraduate pre-medical studies and four years of medical school).

After graduation from medical school at age 26, I then pursued training in Internal Medicine at the University of Michigan, which was a 3-year program where I learned to manage complex problems associated with internal organs, including the heart, lungs, gastrointestinal tract, kidneys, and others. I then went on to pursue an additional 3 years of specialty medical training (fellowship) in the field of gastroenterology. The completion of that program culminated 14 years of post-high school education. It was as that point, at the tender age of 32 and searching for my first job, that I could say that my career in medicine began.

Over that 14-year time period of training, I, and many others like me, made tremendous sacrifices. Only now as I sit with my laptop in the dead of night, with the sounds of my children sleeping, can I look back and see where my journey began.

For me, it began in college, taking rigorous pre-medical courses against a large yearly burden of tuition: $27,000 of debt yearly for 4 years. I was one of the fortunate ones. Because I excelled in a competitive academic environment in high school and was able to maintain a position in the top tier of my class, I obtained an academic scholarship, covering 70% of this tuition. I was fortunate to have graduated from college with "only" $25,000 in student debt. Two weeks after finishing my undergraduate education, I began medical school. After including books, various exams that would typically cost

$1,000-$3,000 per test, and medical school tuition, my yearly education costs amounted to $45,000 per year. Unlike most other fields of study, the demands of medical school education, with daytime classes and night time studying, make it nearly impossible to hold down an extra source of income. I spent an additional $5,000 in my final year for application fees and interview travel as I sought a residency position in internal medicine. After being "matched" into a residency position in Michigan, I took out yet another $10,000 loan to relocate and pay for my final expenses in medical school, as moving expenses are not paid for by training programs.

At that point, with medical school completed, I was only halfway through my journey to becoming a doctor. I recall a moment then, sitting with a group of students in a room with a financial advisor who was saying something about how to consolidate loans. I stared meekly at numbers on a piece of paper listing what I owed for the two degrees that I had earned, knowing full well that I didn't yet have the ability to earn a dime. I didn't know whether to cry at the number or be happy that mine was lower than most of my friends. My number was $196,000.

$196,000. That was the bill for the tuition, the tests, the books, and the late-night pizza. $196,000 financed through a combination of student loans, personal loans, and high-interest credit cards, now consolidated, amalgamated, homogenized into one life-defining number for my personal convenience.

I then relocated to Michigan and moved into a small condo in Ann Arbor, where I started my residency. As a resident in internal medicine, I earned a salary of $39,000. All the while, interest continued to accrue on my motherlode of debt at the rate of $6,000 per year due to the high debt burden. Paying down this debt was not possible while raising two children. My wife began working, but her meager salary as a teacher was barely enough to cover daycare costs. During residency, my costs for taking licensing examinations, interviewing for specialty training positions, and interest on the large loan ballooned my debt further, now exceeding $230,000, all before I began my career as a "real doctor."

Relatives and friends often ask me, "now that you are a 'real' doctor, aren't you making the big bucks?" While I am fortunate to now be making a higher salary, some basics of finance make my salary significantly less than meets the eye (http://drbenbrownmd.wordpress.com/). First, I was 32 years old as I began training and I now had over $230,000 in debt. Had I invested my talents in other pursuits such as law school, I would not have built up this level of debt. Also, as I did not start saving when I was younger, financially speaking, I have lost the past 10 years without the ability to save and invest to earn compounding interest. In addition, as physicians, though we make more money than many others, we are not reimbursed for many of the services that we provide.

We do not "clock" the number of minutes as attorneys do when we talk with patients. We do not hang up the phone as attorneys may do if they are not going to get paid. No, we listen to patients and answer their questions, however long it may take. Even if it is the 32nd straight hour of work, which happens very often, we listen, respond, and formulate a logical plan. If it involves calling a patient at home after I just worked 30 hours in a row and just walked in the door to see my family, I do it. I never come "home" from work. As physicians, we are always available, and have to respond in an intellectual way using the $230,000 rigorous education that we received. And if we don't do our work well, we don't just lose business, but we can lose our livelihood through lawsuits.

You may ask why do we do all of this? It's because we have pride in what we do. We truly care for the well-being of the human race. We have been conditioned to think, act, talk, and work as a very efficient machine, able to handle emotions, different cultures, different ranges of intellect, all to promote the health of America. We are doctors.

In reading this letter, one may think that one has to sacrifice a significant amount to become a great physician. You may think we face physical and mental stress that is unparalleled. You may begin to think that doctors not only have to be smart, but they have to know how to communicate with others during very emotional times. You may think that we must face adversity well and must develop very rough skin to handle all walks of life, especially when dealing with sickness and death on a daily basis.

Now that you see this additional aspect to our career, you may think that we have a tough job to tackle several tasks at once, demanding much versatility. You may think someone needs a great work ethic to do what we do. You must think that not only do we have to know science extremely well, we also have to know other areas such as writing, history, math, even law given the multiple calculations we go through in our heads on a daily basis and conversations we have with families. And finally, you must think we know finance, as we have to try to balance a $230,000 loan while making $50,000 at age 30.

Now imagine, if you would, having $230,000 in debt with two young children at age 30 and listening to the news, with lawmakers saying that doctors are "rich" and should have their pay cut. Or that "studies show that doctors lack empathy."

Unfortunately, we physicians do not have much of a voice on Capitol Hill. There are not enough doctors in Washington, D.C., who can give the insight of this letter while lawmakers in Washington, D.C., discuss healthcare reform. One may hear from leaders of the American Medical Association, but these are not the doctors on the front lines. These are the older political voices who were physicians when the times were different, when doctors did get reimbursed fairly for their work, when student loan debt was not this high, and when lawsuits were less prevalent. Many of the loudest voices in the healthcare debate are those of lawyers and lobbyists for special interests. They do not care about the well-being of patients; that is what doctors do.

I want to make it clear that this letter is not just another story about the difficulties of becoming a doctor and being successful in medicine. I do not want you to think I am complaining about how hard my life is and used to be. In fact, I love my job and there is no other field I would ever imagine myself doing. My true wish is to illustrate the sacrifices doctors do make because I feel we are not represented when laws are made. These sacrifices include a lack of quality family time, our large student loan debt, the age at which we can practically start saving for retirement, and the pressure we face with lawyers watching every move we make. Yet we make these sacrifices gladly for the good of our patients.

I want to challenge our leaders to address the points I have made in this letter, keeping in mind that this is an honest first-hand account of the personal life of a newly practicing physician. It is a letter that speaks for almost all physicians in America and our struggles on our arduous yet personally rewarding life. It is not just a letter of my own journey, but one that represents most physicians' path on our way to caring for America's sick.

You may ask how I had the time to write this letter? As I'm sure many of you do, I made time. It is now 3:00 a.m. on my only day off this month. I considered this a priority. I hope you feel the same. I just finished my 87-hour week. Time for a short rest.

CHAPTER 16

Understanding the Doctors' Reality

THE ARTICLE I SHARED IN THE PREVIOUS CHAPTER was widely circulated and people connected to it from all over the world. It was published or mentioned in many leading news sites, including *The Guardian* and *The Wall Street Journal*, and I appeared on a New York radio talk show to talk about it. However, some people did not relate, wondering how I, as one of the "10%ers," had the nerve to complain.

I intend to respond to that question, but first want to assure everyone that I am not complaining about my job. I am quite content with my job and believe the sacrifices that I made over the past 14 years are well worth it—I love my job and take personal satisfaction in helping my patients. If people read the entire article rather than skimming it and picking out random sentences out of context, they would see that.

One complaint I do have, however, is about the lack of respect doctors receive from a financial and social viewpoint, despite the rigors of training and the complexity of our work as described in this book. The other issue relates to the *future* of doctors' salaries, not our current salaries. Lawmakers think that doctors, especially primary care doctors, can absorb cuts in the future. Cuts to doctors' pay are likely and we have already seen cuts over the past 10 years. We have seen a 20% cut to our fees already in the past 15 years. Other businesses cannot absorb 4% cuts, let alone 20% cuts, as their expenses will exceed their revenue. Lawmakers need to understand where doctors in general are coming from since we do not have "everyday" doctors speaking to lawmakers. And this is what this book illustrates.

In addition to the above points, my article was speaking for all doctors, not just gastroenterologists. The average internal medicine doctor makes $170,000 and the average pediatrician makes $140,000, but remember, doctors don't begin earning that income—much less putting money away in savings—until they are in their mid-30s. Most Americans have the opportunity to start saving in their early 20s, assuming they get a bachelor's degree. When doctors are in their 20s, they don't have income. The stipend in residency translates to about $9/hour for six years of post-med school training.

When considering the point I am trying to make, please see Dr. Ben Brown's article in which he illustrates how doctors make as much per hour as a public school teacher despite 10 extra years of training (www. benbrownmd.wordpress.com). It translates to less than the current minimum wage in some states! We assume that a physician makes $200,000/year and a teacher makes $60,000/year. However, after accounting for zero income for four years in medical school, 80+ hours of work for the physician for three years of residency, and the fact that the physician was making $35,000 per year while working 80 hours per week (no overtime pay), one can see how the average hourly wage comes out to $8.41, which is less than minimum wage!

In addition, when one adds to that the $190,000 debt a doctor has to pay off over the years and the loss of compounding interest over those seven years of medical school and residency training, one realizes that the salaries of teachers and doctors are similar despite the physician's seven extra years of training/schooling.

Compounding interest is the main way to develop wealth. Even Warren Buffett stated that the three factors that contributed to his wealth were 1) being born in America, 2) living a long time, and 3) compounding interest. Specialists finish training at age 33. We lost 11 years of compounding interest compared to the average 22-year-old college graduate. By losing those years and having to defer savings, I need to save thousands of dollars more per year than if I started saving when I was 22 years old. I may have a high income, but I am in no way wealthy.

Unfair Tax Laws and a Salary Well-Earned

When we do eventually make more money (12 years later than the average person who gets a bachelor's degree), the tax laws negatively affect us on many fronts. First and most obvious, we cannot write off our student loan interest. Despite accruing $196,000 at 2.8% interest, I cannot write off the $6,000 per year I pay in interest. The point of the tax law was to provide relief to students, but because our income is naturally higher after training based on IRS limits, we cannot write our student loan interest off. Yes, the people who need this relief the most are the ones who are exempt from this benefit. It's a similar scenario with rental home losses. Despite me trying to be responsible and not short sell my condo, I cannot write off my rental losses on my tax return due to IRS income limits. We are taxed at a very high tax bracket just because we have a high income, not because we have real wealth. In fact, I have no wealth. I have an income that I am taxed upon heavily and have $196,000 worth of debt.

This is why it is frustrating when people say, "You're a rich doctor." I am not a rich or wealthy doctor. I am a doctor with a high income compared to America's median salary, but I also have 10 times as much debt as the average American. And I lost the advantage of compounding interest, a huge factor that allows wealth in America. And I am taxed heavily due to my high income. I have a high income, but no wealth. There is a huge difference, which I describe later in this next chapter.

Yes, we have loads of debt that accrues interest, which prohibits even more savings. While the business graduate is saving $1,000/month at age 33 and already saved in his 20s, I am paying off a loan at $1,400/month with no savings. Plus, I need to save even more than others my age now because I was not able to in my 20s. Saving can be hard when one has kids and 40% percent of one's income is lost to taxes because one is in a high tax bracket. So basically, instead of being able to save $1,400/month for retirement, I am paying that much per month on a large loan. Where is the money that I can actually save after accounting for all these negative laws?

I did not mention other unfair tax laws such as the phase outs for personal exemptions and itemized deductions. Basically, because I make more money now, I cannot use exemptions for having kids. Kids cost money no matter how much one makes. And add to that a $190,000 debt load and I feel as if I cannot afford much at all despite a respectable income. The other unfair aspects include paying for our multiple board exams, which each cost at least $1,000, and paying our own way for interviews, even though we have no income in medical school. Where do people think this money comes from? Unless that medical student has parents or relatives who can afford this, this money comes in the form of more loans and unsecured debt. Not only is tuition for medical school expensive, but add in the required exams, books, and interview travel, and we are adding a whole new financial dimension.

If one knew the sacrifices we had to make on this journey, one would realize that a large salary at the end of 14 years of post-high school training is reasonable. We don't just leave work at 6:00 p.m. If patients' families have questions, we stay as long it takes to help that patient. For example, the other day, I was talking to a hospital patient and his son about his bile duct cancer diagnosis. This conversation usually lasts 30 minutes or so, as the prognosis is poor. About 25 minutes into the conversation, another family member entered the room and I basically had to reiterate everything I had just discussed, including drawing diagrams about the diagnosis. And of course, during this time, I got paged about another patient issue.

My wife has lived through 10 years of hearing me say, "I'll be home in 20 minutes," only to see me walk in the door two hours later. We are not getting paid for these hours spent talking to families. We do not clock out of work. We did 33-hour shifts in residency (working more than 90 hours/week for three years) and took call every fourth night. Even after training, we wake up at 2:00 a.m. to drive into the city to help patients, answer calls off hours, and do not clock minutes like lawyers do.

What's more, we have people's lives in our hands. We are sedating patients using powerful medicines, and performing life-saving, yet risky procedures on a nightly basis. We have to remove razor blades from a suicidal patient's stomach, or urgently cut off the blood supply so a patient does not bleed to death. These are not simple chores like fixing a clogged toilet. If we make a mistake, the consequence can be a lengthy hospitalization or death or a multi-million-dollar suit against us. If my plumber messes up, I cannot sue him. He simply comes back and repairs the problem. If my mortgage lender messes up my mortgage, I don't sue him. And his job is not high risk to begin with. He is selling a loan over the phone, not sedating and performing life-saving procedures. But we are doctors; we can handle it.

Most doctors studied their hearts out since high school, worked their tails off in medical school and residency, and were likely in the top 10% every step along the way from high school through college. They were studying while their friends were playing football in the backyard. They were studying while their friends went to frat parties. They were studying at home while their friends took family vacations.

Given the high risk involved in our jobs, the risk we put on our own health (sleepless nights, high stress), the sacrifices we made to get through four years of medical school and six years of 90-hour work weeks, and the desire to persist despite being $200,000 in debt while making $10/hour in residency, don't you think we deserve what we get? If you don't understand this or think this is an entitled attitude, then I challenge you to complete the required training and then speak up in about 10 years (assuming you have a bachelor's degree). It is easy to skim an article with your morning coffee and think, "I could've done this." It is easy to say, "I can stay up all night if I have to." Well, try staying up for 33 hours, then trying to recite histories on complex patients or perform intensive procedures while having a patient's life in your hands. It's one thing to think it; it is another to actually live it and experience it, with all its pain, suffering, and triumph.

Income versus Wealth—A Huge Difference

It is also easy to say, "Boy, doctors make so much. It must be nice to be able to afford nice cars." Let me respond to this all-too-common declaration through examples. There is a huge difference between being wealthy (rich) and having a high income. ***High incomes do not correlate with wealth.***

An article by the Cato Institute's Richard W. Rahn, who is a senior fellow of the Cato Institute (a public policy research organization), appeared as a commentary in the *Washington Times* on August 27, 2008 (www.cato.org/publications/commentary/confusing-wealth-income) and sums up this wealth-versus-income debate well:

> Which of the following families is "richer"? The first family consists of a wife who has recently become a medical doctor, and she makes $160,000 per year. Her husband is a small business entrepreneur who makes $110,000 per year, giving them a total family income of $270,000 per year. However, they are still paying off the loans the wife took out for medical school and the loans the husband took out to start his business, amounting to debts of $300,000. Their total assets are valued at $450,000; hence, their real net worth or wealth (the difference between gross assets and liabilities) is only $150,000.
>
> The second family consists of a trial lawyer who took early retirement and his non-working wife. They have an annual income of $230,000, all of it derived from interest on tax-free municipal bonds they own. However, their net worth is $7 million,

consisting of $5 million in bonds, a million-dollar home with no mortgage, and a million dollars in art work, home furnishings, automobiles and personal items.

The second family is clearly far better off financially than the first family, yet many in the U.S. Congress, including Sen. Barack Obama, want to increase taxes on the first (and poorer) family and not on the wealthier family. They have mis-defined "rich" by confusing a flow (income) with a stock (real net assets), and thus come to the wrong conclusion. They want to tax those (who make more than $250,000 a year) who are trying to become rich, while preserving the status for those who already have wealth.

Increasing taxes on those 2.3 million American households who earn more than $250,000 per year is foolish and destructive for several reasons. It reduces the incentives for highly productive people to spend years in school obtaining needed skills, and then work hard in producing goods and services desired by their fellow citizens. It encourages the misallocation of productive resources by encouraging people to find ways to minimize the tax burden rather than to use their labor and savings for the highest and best use. It reduces the mobility of families up and down the income scale, and freezes the advantages of those who have substantial inherited wealth (e.g., the Kennedys, Kerrys, Pelosis, etc.).

Those who want the "rich" to pay more or "give back" not only confuse income with wealth, but also fail to understand life cycle mobility, and the effects of taxation and income redistribution programs on "disposable income." Many people, when they are young (including the average graduate student), would be classified as poor in terms of taxable income. Most people have a sharp rise in family or "household" income after they graduate from school, and many of these enter the definition of "upper income" in their forties and fifties, but after they retire, their taxable income often drops to the point where they are considered middle income, even though they may have more than a million dollars in net assets. Income distribution is most often defined by "household" income as contrasted with individual income. Most low-income "households" consist of single (often young) individuals, while most families with more than one income earner are higher income "households." The fact is there are about four times as many households (8.9 million) that have net assets of a million or more than there are households that earn more than $250,000. And many of the high-income households do not have a million dollars in net assets.

Many politicians and media people confuse taxable income with disposable and in-kind income. Because of the highly progressive income tax system, (97 percent of income taxes are paid by the top 50 percent of income earners and the top 1 percent pays 40 percent of the tax, despite having only 20 percent of the income), the difference in high-income and low-income families in after-tax income is far less than pre-tax income. In addition, there are many government welfare and subsidy programs for low-income people that are not included in many of the standard definitions of income.

Given that high marginal tax rates on income are counterproductive, some have argued for a wealth tax, but that doesn't work either. A wealth tax mainly taxes productive capital, thus reducing job and productivity growth, and it also encourages people to move their wealth to other countries and/or engage in extravagant expenditures—as the French have found out, much to their regret.

Those who confuse taxable income with wealth are guilty of both sloppy use of language and sloppy thinking. Is it prudent to trust the writing of the tax code to a group of sloppy thinkers?

This article really drives home this point. Stop making a villain of someone who has earned a high income through years of school and 14 years of very rigorous training. There is always a story behind it and my story is the story in the example of the family with a high income, but no wealth. So stop calling doctors who have earned their way to a higher than average income rich or wealthy. If calling a doctor with $230,000 in debt with no savings and a $150,000 mortgage wealthy or rich, then you missed the point.

Misconceptions of Doctors Reimbursement

My grandmother once commented, "Matt, if you get paid $2,000 to do a colonoscopy for 30 minutes, you must be rich." Like many people, my grandmother misunderstands how doctors are paid. The way doctors currently are reimbursed is unique to the medical profession. The charges that patients see on their bills do not represent the amount doctors are paid. These are inflated numbers derived from contracts between hospitals and insurance companies. When a hospital or doctor submits a charge (bill), the insurance companies or Medicare/Medicaid, depending on the patient's insurance, use a fee schedule that consists of thousands of codes that assign dollar amounts for individual procedures or clinic visits (available on the American Medical Association website: www.ama-assn.org). Each code has a dollar figure and a relative value unit (RVU) to determine how much to reimburse that doctor. This is called a "Medicare fee schedule." Insurance companies will pay a certain percentage of the fee based on Medicare. So when hospital groups negotiate with insurance companies such as Blue Cross or Aetna, they negotiate what percentage of Medicare they will pay the doctor and the hospital. This can range from 80% to 180% of Medicare, depending on the insurance carrier.

If a patient has Medicare, however, one can see exactly what that doctor will get paid based on the CPT (current procedural terminology) code (it varies 1% based on geography) by using the fee schedule. Each procedure or office visit is assigned a CPT code. This is often called the "allowable charge" on patients' bills. The revenue (not net income) the doctor receives is in fact this fee (not the charge) and is set no matter how much the hospital or doctor chooses to charge.

To complicate matters, there usually are two different charges in a patient's bill: a "professional" charge from the doctor, and a "facility" or "hospital" charge (an inflated charge that goes to the facility or the hospital, not the doctor). If he or she works for a hospital, the doctor sees only the professional charge, not the hospital charge. The professional charge is the charge for the doctors' services, such as office visit, procedure, or MRI interpretation. The doctor receives only a fraction of this professional charge because it is reduced by the fee schedule to the appropriate amount. In the end, a doctor sees only a small fraction of the original charge (the bill the patient may see) and this does not include overhead expenses the practice incurs, which can range from 30% to 60%.

Let's go back to my grandmother's example. The overall charge, which includes the facility charge and the professional charge, was $2,500. That's the amount she saw on the bill. Breaking that down, the professional (doctor) charge was $700, but the doctor only got reimbursed (paid) $202 for that colonoscopy based on the Medicare fee schedule. And assuming the doctor has a 50% overhead to the practice, he or she was actually paid about $100 for that colonoscopy. And that is assuming the insurance company or the patient pays the doctor. That's less than a plumber gets paid for the service call and one hour of work on your toilet. No offense to plumbers, but that plumber didn't go to school for 14 years, is not preventing colon cancer, and is not sedating a live human being with a risk of causing great bodily harm, even death.

Our government leaders don't understand this system any more than the public. In a healthcare town hall meeting in New Hampshire, President Obama claimed that surgeons get paid (not charged) "$30,000 to $50,000" for a foot amputation (www.youtube.com/watch?v=rIVieMfb2SI). Looking at the Medicare fee schedule, CPT code 28805 states that the surgeon would get paid $738.90, which is the fee before his or her office expenses are considered, including office space, staffing, and medical liability. Thus, the doctor actually gets paid 1.4% of what President Obama claimed he is paid.

Doctors' payment systems are confusing for patients and create much anxiety. They apparently also are confusing to lawmakers who are trying to modify reimbursement without understanding the system. Doctors can charge whatever they want, but what they actually are paid is out of their hands.

In addition, if a procedure takes longer than average or is more complex, a doctor is not paid more for that procedure—there is no overtime or extra pay if the procedure is more difficult than expected. The fee is pre-determined by the Medicare fee schedule no matter how sick the patient is. There is no extra charge if the procedure is done after hours or on a weekend. In addition, if there is a follow-up call and three family members want to discuss results, this is part of the one fee; no additional fees are billed. We do not get paid for emails or phone calls even though we often spend five times the amount of time on the phone as a lawyer may. If a patient arrives late and needs to talk for 30 minutes versus 15 minutes, we give them that time and we do not get paid additional fees.

This is unmistakably different for other professionals. Lawyers for example, can bill a client for a letter or fax associated with their case. They can bill for engaging in small talk before a meeting. I cannot charge for talking to a sick patient at 2:00 a.m., even if that conversation lasts 30 minutes and I have a full work schedule the next day.

I am not criticizing the way lawyers get paid; I simply am stating that lawyers and doctors bill in very different ways, and sometimes this difference is not noticed. I speak with patients in the middle of the night and I spend the extra 30 minutes helping patients get the quality care they deserve because I went into medicine to help those in need and I get satisfaction from this. I do worry, however, that this may not continue to be the case for all doctors if reimbursement models are not modified and doctors' fees are not corrected for inflation and practice expenses. They simply will not bring in enough revenue to cover their expenses. We already are seeing a trend toward concierge medicine due to decreasing reimbursement and higher costs. Concierge medicine is a practice in which patients are charged a yearly fee by the doctor to have easier access to the doctor they sign a contract with. It eliminates the need to wait, and more personalized attention is given. Unfortunately, this idea will cause costs to be passed on to patients.

Doctors have a calling to help human beings and we take this seriously. However, Capitol Hill needs doctors from the front lines to discuss our issues so that the best reform decisions possible can be made. Doctors should not be afraid or ashamed to bring these issues up. It is only by logical thoughtful discussion can Americans move forward. We owe this to ourselves and to the millions of people who look to doctors to treat their ailments. Congress must seek out practicing doctors (not lobbyists or lawmakers) with experience on the front lines of care to help them arrive at a fair system that can benefit everyone.

We need this to preserve world-class healthcare system and to keep our citizens healthy. That is my hope.

Why Aren't Doctors Involved in the Healthcare Reform Process?

As I was watching CNN news recently, the discussion turned to different ways the Affordable Care Act (ACA) is failing, including high-deductible plans (up to $12,700 for families), substandard insurance plans, and loss of current insurance plans due to the ACA. One patient complained, "My new healthcare plan tripled in price, and now it's like having a third loan to deal with, including my car and home loan." A vicious cycle of blame between

Washington, health insurance companies, and the patients is quickly demoralizing this nation and increasing costs and administrative regulations.

Surprisingly, doctors were not part of the discussion—as if doctors don't know the intricacies of how the healthcare system works. As if doctors are not there for their patients 24 hours per day, ordering tests or doing procedures that can benefit a patient's well-being. As if doctors are not dealing with denials from the insurance companies on a daily basis, losing valuable hours to menial paperwork that could be spent caring for our nation's sick.

Doctors have a duty to care for their patients and are the engines that put healthcare into motion. They yearn to maintain that physician-patient relationship that is important to the well-being of our patients. Unfortunately, doctors are not being directly involved in the healthcare reform even though they would provide valuable insight into the day-to-day operations of this healthcare machine.

Would you want to fly in a plane with no input from a pilot? Or design a curriculum without a teacher's input? These "insider" insights are essential to healthcare in order to exact true change and improve healthcare for everyone. Unless we embrace this idea and look to doctors to help solve these dilemmas, we will be doomed with increasing prices, more talking heads on TV blaming others, and dysfunctional insurance companies who have never spent a minute shadowing a doctor, yet claiming to have all the answers.

The current law and regulations being implemented under the Affordable Care Act will ultimately lead to sicker patients and lower quality care for three reasons:

1. Older doctors will retire early, fed up with the system. These older doctors believe the loss of a patient-physician relationship and the burdensome regulations (paperwork) will choke off their ability to provide good care. In addition, their expenses are increasing with these new regulations. Add in the projected cuts in reimbursement up to 26%, and their livelihood will be threatened (http://money.cnn.com/2013/11/01/news/economy/ medicare-doctor-payments). These cuts could force these doctors out of practice or force them to stop seeing Medicare patients simply because their expenses (which increase yearly) are exceeding their declining reimbursement, which has declined steadily over the past several years.

2. Smart young minds will no longer enter the field due to rising debt (average $250,000 after medical school) and yearly threats of 26% cuts to

reimbursement. When young college students realize after going to school and training for 14 years that they cannot provide for a family in the face of $250,000 in medical school debt and deferred income for all those years, they will turn to different professions (www.moneynews.com/InvestingAnalysis/Medical-School-Bernanke-Son-Debt/2013/04/11/id/498930/).

3. Today's younger doctors will become more demoralized with administration and lawmakers dictating how they provide care. They will feel as if they are increasingly being treated as machines, expecting to provide great care such as answering patient calls at 2:00 a.m., working 24-hour shifts, doing more procedures for less, and filling out more and more paperwork, all with the threat of being sued if they don't perform without making a mistake. This will produce a high burnout rate and poorer care. Here is an article posted on KevinMD.com (www.kevinmd.com/blog/2014/12/confessions-burnt-physician.html) from a doctor (anonymous) who recently left medicine due to burn out:

> I've wanted to be a physician for as long as I can remember. As a teen, the choice to become a doctor seemed to perfectly meld my affinity for science, academics and helping others. Better yet, pediatrics offered the ability to work with families and children of all ages and developmental abilities.
>
> For fifteen years, I lived, breathed, and worked toward my goal to become a pediatrician. In college, I studied the foundational cornerstones of science and humanities and focused on how health impacts the rest of our lives. In medical school, I learned about different aspects of each organ system and marveled at the miracles of the human body. During residency, I walked the halls of hospitals during the wee hours of the morning. I rubbed the sleep out of my eyes as I provided artificial breaths to a dying infant and smoothed the crinkles in my yellowing white coat as we brainstormed why another child was brought to us at death's door.
>
> When I finally achieved my goal to call myself a board-certified pediatrician, I beamed as I walked into my new office space that had my name posted on the wall outside exam room doors.

Despite my lofty dreams and expectations, practicing primary care pediatrics was nothing like I hoped it would be. My days were filled with opportunities to meet and grow with patients and families, but my tidbits of time were sliced into 15-minute increments. As my practice size increased, I was persistently pressured to add extra patients over my lunch hours before the day started, and into time slots already booked with other patients. The need to move increasingly efficiently sparked anxiety within me. I was halfway through greeting one patient before I was also surreptitiously listening for the opening and closing of the next exam room door to signal that another patient was waiting.

The physical and emotional work of completing a visit every 15 minutes repeatedly refreshing my smile before I burst into the next room began to make me feel like a machine. As a robot in the factory of medicine, the demands of my job pulled at my greatest skills of empathy and compassion, two of the character traits that made me most suited for primary care. Try as I might, it was hard to feel compassionate for the mother of a child with a mild cold when I was already ignoring my raging headache, need to urinate, and fatigue. Despite my gut instinct to address the 'one last thing' that patients often bring up at the end of a visit, the pressure of metrics that detailed my length of visit and wait time for patients coerced me to ignore their concerns, even if my actions translated into another office visit, another co-pay, another day.

When I did have time to sit down, I was crowded into the corner of a small office shared by two other physicians. When we all were present and trying to make phone calls, type office notes, and converse with staff, the cacophony rose. My brain and my inner self were desperate for peace, though I knew it would be only moments before the next patient was ready in a room to begin again.

By the time I got home each evening, I was a deflated emotional balloon, sucked of energy and ambition and left with little to share. When my own children rushed to greet me, I offered them a quick hug and kiss and then silently wished they would quiet down. After dinner and bedtime stories, I rested with them until it was time to open my laptop again and work through additional charts, emails, and work tasks. My husband personified my laptop as a bedfellow in our marriage. I struggled for the emotional energy to make my steadfast lifetime partner feel loved.

As a part of the middle management administration at my healthcare organization, I sat in meetings week after week where the physicians in the organization were referred to as "lazy, whiny, irresponsible, and unmotivated." I gazed through the picturesque windows in the large administrative offices and chuckled at the irony that money is too tight to upgrade or expand space in clinics to improve the workplace environment. I seethed quietly as I listened to the mantra that we need to see more patients, more efficiently, and work longer hours as if I were listening to the drumbeat at a funeral march.

The articles on physician burnout cite the need for physicians to develop coping strategies to deal with the daily stressors incurred in the office. We are tasked to learn and practice mindfulness, meditation, and regular exercise. While I make exercise a priority, I simply can't find the time to learn the other soul-saving techniques in my current work environment. I think it is not only a physician's responsibility to take care of ourselves, but the scaffolding of the healthcare system needs allow for practices that will sustain those of us at its very core.

Last week, I submitted my resignation from medicine.

Many have asked me if I will ever come back, but I'm not sure. I am jaded by the push to provide efficient and effective healthcare for others while ignoring my own personal needs. I am saddened by the palpable wounds that I have left my children through lack of energy, lack of engagement, and inability to be there when they need me. I am discouraged that despite 15 years of focus and sacrifice, Dr. Google has become a smarter and more esteemed physician than I. I am worried that the advent and elevation of pseudoscience has led to increased vaccine resistance, re-emergence of previously eradicated diseases, and hours of time spent fruitlessly discussing why the opinions of thousand physician researchers should outweigh the thoughts of one or two dissenters.

I have heard that it costs up to $10,000 every time my organization hires and trains a new physician. It costs patients and insurance companies each time I ask a patient come back to discuss other concerns I didn't have time to address. Every time I order a diagnostic test that is not medically warranted, but desired by a patient that has Googled their symptoms, costs increase.

The United States spent approximately $8,895 per person for healthcare in 2012, which is higher than any other developed country but is among the worst health outcomes. If we want to decrease the cost of American healthcare, it will be imperative to make efforts to retain primary care physicians, decrease administrative costs and overhead spending, and put back some autonomy in physician's hands so that customer satisfaction does not override the importance of good patient care. In addition, healthcare companies and patients need to recognize that those of us who chose to study medicine are not merely well-trained machines but humans who strive to deliver care with compassion, empathy, and expertise.

I don't know what my next career will be, but for now I will work on regaining what made me choose medicine in the first place. As I cultivate the human that has been suppressed by the robot that provided medical care, I look forward to regaining the health and happiness that we seek for all.

These doctors went into medicine to feel a healthy bond between themselves and their patients. They enjoy talking and spending time with them in the office. Doctors want autonomy because treating patients involves nuances administrators don't understand. We should not be judged by patient satisfaction scores. Recently, patient satisfaction scores have become more common in healthcare systems. They usually are tied to the doctor's compensation in that his or her pay gets docked if he or she doesn't meet a certain threshold in terms of patient satisfaction. While providing great service is important and not denying the fact that there are doctors with very poor bedside manner, I and almost all of my doctor colleagues challenge these satisfaction scores as inaccurate and unfounded.

The industry wants to make patients become customers who can demand a service. The major problem is that patients are not customers. Customers buy nice dinners, condos, or cars. When they buy these goods or services, they expect something nice because they are voluntarily doing these actions. When one gets sick, one is not a customer, but rather a patient. Patients are not on vacation. They are not in the mood to be at the doctor's office. They do not want to be there. They have not chosen to have this service. Rather, they are sick and want to feel better. In addition, patients are not buying a product, demanding a good outcome. When you go to a resort, you expect to have a lovely vacation. At a doctor's office, the outcome may be grim. How can patients be satisfied if they just were diagnosed with a cancer or if their chronic abdominal pain was not "fixed" in a 30-minute office visit? Patient care is not about being happy and satisfied. It is about delivering quality care, which all too often is not good news.

Finally, doctors with high patient satisfaction scores are not necessarily better doctors. According to a national study published in the March 2012 *Archives of Internal Medicine* (www.ncbi.nlm.nih.gov/pubmed/22331982), higher patient satisfaction was associated with higher healthcare use and increased mortality. Hospitals have been trying to promote a business model of patient satisfaction by making patients customers. But let's face it: patients aren't customers. They are sick and they want to feel better. When doctors get bad customer service scores because "the walls in the office did not match" or "it took too long to check in," they are being judged not on their skill, but on the patient's subjective opinion about something totally unrelated to his or her care.

This kind of administrative control is what breaks doctors down and discourages them. They are being told what to do by administrators who have never stepped foot into a medical school and have never seen a sick patient in the office. We are not to be judged by how a patient's blood sugars are controlled. These are black and white measures that administrators come up with to make medicine a business. These measures are conjured up by administrators to increase profits, not to benefit a patient's well-being.

Medicine is an intimate, personal relationship with another human being who is vulnerable. It is not a business.

Unfortunately, with all the unnecessary documentation, regulations and time restraints, doctors are losing the bond that is so critical for care. They are becoming cogs in the wheel, labeled not as doctors, but rather as "health-care providers." Those doctors who choose to stay in the field of medicine may elect to practice concierge medicine, taking the insurance company and hospital administrators out of the equation and attempting to maintain the physician-patient relationship. With current doctors feeling demoralized and younger students afraid to enter the field, we will see a massive shortage of doctors that will threaten the health of our citizens.

An article written by Robert Gunderson on September 26, 2014, entitled "How Hospitals Discourage Doctors," perfectly sums up how many doctors feel about the increasing demands from administration:

> Not accustomed to visiting hospital executive suites, I took my seat in the waiting room somewhat warily.
>
> Seated across from me was a handsome man in a well-tailored three-piece suit, whose thoroughly professional appearance made me—in my rumpled white coat, sheaves of dog-eared paper bulging from both pockets—feel out of place.
>
> Within a minute, an administrative secretary came out and escorted him into one of the offices. Exhausted from a long call shift and lulled by the quiet, I started to doze off. Soon roused by the sound of my own snoring, I started and looked about.
>
> That was when I spotted the document on an adjacent chair. Its title immediately caught my eye: "How to Discourage a Doctor."
>
> No one else was about, so I reached over, picked it up, and began to leaf through its pages. It became apparent immediately that it was one of the most remarkable things I had ever read, clearly not meant for my eyes. It seemed to be the product of a health care consulting company, presumably the well-dressed man's employer. Fearing that he would return any moment to retrieve it, I perused it as quickly as possible. My recollection of its contents is naturally somewhat imperfect, but I can reproduce the gist of what it said:

The stresses on today's hospital executive are enormous. They include a rapidly shifting regulatory environment, downward pressures on reimbursement rates, and seismic shifts in payment mechanisms. Many leaders naturally feel as though they are building a hospital in the midst of an earthquake. With prospects for revenue enhancement highly uncertain, the best strategy for ensuring a favorable bottom line is to reduce costs. And for the foreseeable future, the most important driver of costs in virtually every hospital will be its medical staff.

Though physician compensation accounts for only about 8% of health care spending, decisions that physicians strongly influence or make directly—such as what medication to prescribe, whether to perform surgery, and when to admit and discharge a patient from the hospital—have been estimated to account for as much as 80% of the nation's health care budget. To maintain a favorable balance sheet, hospital executives need to gain control of their physicians. Most hospitals have already taken an important step in this direction by employing a growing proportion of their medical staff.

Transforming previously independent physicians into employees has increased hospital influence over their decision making, an effect that has been successfully augmented in many centers by tying physician compensation directly to the execution of hospital strategic initiatives. But physicians have invested many years in learning their craft, they hold their professional autonomy in high esteem, and they take seriously the considerable respect and trust with which many patients still regard them.

As a result, the challenge of managing a hospital medical staff continues to resemble herding cats.

Merely controlling the purse strings is not enough. To truly seize the reins of medicine, it is necessary to do more, to get into the heads and hearts of physicians. And the way to do this is to show physicians that they are not nearly so important as they think they are. Physicians have long seen the patient-physician relationship as the very center of the health care solar system. As we go forward, they must be made to feel that this relationship is not the sun around which everything else orbits, but rather one of the dimmer peripheral planets, a Neptune or perhaps Uranus.

How can this goal be achieved? A complete list of proven tactics and strategies is available to our clients, but some of the more notable include the following:

Make health care incomprehensible to physicians. It is no easy task to baffle the most intelligent people in the organization, but it can be done. For example, make physicians increasingly dependent on complex systems outside their domain of expertise, such as information technology and coding and billing software. Ensure that such systems are very costly, so that solo practitioners and small groups, who naturally cannot afford them, must turn to the hospital. And augment their sense of incompetence by making such systems user-unfriendly and unreliable. Where possible, change vendors frequently.

Promote a sense of insecurity among the medical staff. A comfortable physician is a confident physician, and a confident physician usually proves difficult to control. To undermine confidence, let it be known that physicians' jobs are in jeopardy and their compensation is likely to decline. Fire one or more physicians, ensuring that the entire medical staff knows about it. Hire replacements with a minimum of fanfare. Place a significant percentage of compensation at risk, so that physicians begin to feel beholden to hospital administration for what they manage to eke out.

Transform physicians from decision makers to decision implementers. Convince them that their professional judgment regarding particular patients no longer constitutes a reliable compass.

Refer to such decisions as anecdotal, idiosyncratic, or simply insufficiently evidence-based. Make them feel that their mission is not to balance benefits and risks against their knowledge of particular patients, but instead to apply broad practice guidelines to the care of all patients. Hiring, firing, promotion, and all rewards should be based on conformity to hospital-mandated policies and procedures.

Subject physicians to escalating productivity expectations. Borrow terminology and methods from the manufacturing industry to make them think of themselves as production-line workers, then convince them that they are not working sufficiently hard and fast. Show them industry standards and benchmarks in comparison to which their output is subpar. On the off chance that their productivity compares favorably, cite numerous reasons that such benchmarks are biased and move the bar progressively higher.

Increase physicians' responsibility while decreasing their authority. For example, hold physicians responsible for patient satisfaction scores, but ensure that such scores are influenced by a variety of factors over which physicians have little or no control, such as information technology, hospitality of staff members, and parking. The goal of such measures is to induce a state that psychologists refer to as learned helplessness, a growing sense among physicians that whatever they do, they cannot meaningfully influence health care, which is to say the operations of the hospital.

Above all, introduce barriers between physicians and their patients. The more directly physicians and patients feel connected to one another, the greater the threat to the hospital's control. When physicians think about the work they do, the first image that comes to mind should be the hospital, and when patients realize they need care, they should turn first to the hospital, not a particular physician. One effective technique is to ensure that patient-physician relationships are frequently disrupted so that the hospital remains the one constant. Another is . . . .

The sound of a door roused me again. The man in the three-piece suit emerged from the office, he and the hospital executive to whom he had been speaking shaking hands and smiling. As he turned, I looked about. Where was "How to Discourage a Doctor?" It was not on the table, nor was it on the chair where I had first found it. "Will he think I took it?" I wondered. But instead of stopping to look for it, he simply walked out of the office. As I watched him go, one thing became clear: Having read that document, I suddenly felt a lot less discouraged.

I do not want this to continue to happen. I went into medicine as a calling to help others and I take this role seriously. I wanted to sit down and talk with my patients, share stories with them, not on the clock, and without cumbersome, slow computers and administrators documenting every move I make. I want every person in America to have access to quality healthcare at a reasonable price because our citizens deserve this.

Unfortunately, universal access to care at a reasonable price cannot be realized unless lawmakers look to doctors on the front lines of care for specific input. We as doctors know why costs are high and why the public is unfortunately misinformed about how it all works. But we need a representative sample of practicing doctors in Congress discussing these issues so that these "insider" insights can be applied to our current laws.

CHAPTER 17

Ideas That Would Lead to Better and More Affordable Healthcare from a Doctor's Perspective

T HE IDEAS OUTLINED BELOW WOULD LEAD to better and more affordable care.

1. Simplify costs and reimbursement and make them more transparent. These changes would help clarify misconceptions about doctor's pay. Leaders need to stop attacking doctors for how much they earn because they do not really know how it works. In all other professions, one gets paid what the bill says. If a handyman comes in to fix your sink and charges $80, you pay him $80. If a lawyer says he charges $250/hour and he works four hours for you, you owe him $1,000.

Unfortunately, the medical billing system is unique, confusing, and wrong. The charges (bills) that patients see in the mail are not what doctors get paid. These are inflated numbers derived from contracts between hospitals or groups and insurance companies as I discussed earlier in this book. A recent *New York Times* article headline read "As Hospital Prices Soar, a Stitch Costs $500" (www.nytimes.com/2013/12/03/health/as-hospital-costs-soar-single-stitch-tops-500.html?_r=1&). Sadly, these inflated numbers have nothing to do with what the doctor gets paid. In fact, those bills do not go to the doctor at all, but rather to the hospital. I explained these issues about charges versus how much the doctor actually collects earlier in the book.

Another example of confusing costs of medical treatment hits closer to home. My mother presented to the ER with sudden blurry vision a few weeks ago. Several tests were run to rule out causes such as stroke or tumor. Thankfully, her diagnosis was nothing life-threatening and she is recovering. Two weeks later, she received the bill in the mail explaining her charges.

She was shocked at how high the charges were and could not decipher this bill. Referring to my explanations above, under "professional/physician charges," it "appears" a physician gets paid $450 to interpret a CT head and $580 to interpret an MRI of the brain. As I described earlier, this is far from the truth. Looking at the fee schedule, code 70450, a CT head would pay a doctor $29 for a Medicare patient. This is far different than the $450 shown on the bill. In fact, it is only 6% of what the bill states! Likewise, an MRI brain, code 70558, would pay a radiologist $109—way off from the charge of $580. There are other inflated fees for the hospital as you can see in this bill totaling over $11,000, but these are not related to a doctor's compensation.

This clearly illustrates that doctors' payment systems are confusing for patients and create much anxiety when trying to decipher a bill. It is apparently even confusing to lawmakers and to the president, who are trying to modify reimbursement yet do not understand how doctors get paid. Even though a stitch may cost $500, the doctor got paid $28 dollars to read a complex CT scan of the brain. This idea is preposterous. We need real costs to healthcare, not inflated charges from hospitals. This needs to be addressed so patients and lawmakers can understand where doctors are coming from and realize that doctors are getting paid much less than it appears. These bills should be transparent so patients know exactly how much the doctor is getting paid, the same way we know how much a plumber gets paid when he fixes a toilet.

Doctors do not collect whatever they want for clinic visits or procedures; this is all determined by the fee schedule explained above. In addition, if one procedure takes longer than average or is more complex, a doctor does not collect more for that procedure, unlike other professions that are paid hourly. The fee is pre-determined by the Medicare fee schedule no matter how sick the patient is. This fee is standard whether the procedure is performed during business hours or at 3:00 a.m. This is clearly different than other professions that charge an hourly rate.

In addition, if there is a follow-up call or letter after the procedure, this is all part of the one fee and no additional fees are billed. If that patient calls at 9:00 p.m. that night with a health complaint or the patient arrives 30 minutes late to an appointment, there is not an increased charge (i.e., we do not get paid more). I am not suggesting that hourly rate-work is wrong; I am simply stating that work is very different and sometimes this contrast is not noticed.

I speak with patients at 9:00 p.m. and I spend the extra 30 minutes helping patients get the quality care they deserve without extra compensation.

Of course, I do this willingly because I went into medicine to help those in need and I get satisfaction from this. I do worry, however, that this may not continue to be the case for all doctors if reimbursement models are not modified and doctors' fees are not corrected for inflation and practice expenses. Doctors simply will not bring in enough revenue to cover their expenses. Again, doctors' fees have been declining, are not secure, and do not adjust for inflation. Possible solutions involve making costs and charges more transparent and realizing the true (not inflated) costs and benefits of medical devices, services, and materials. With actual costs available and transparent, patients would be given choices and autonomy about their health.

The vehicle for this would be health savings accounts (which I describe in more detail below), which allow patients to use their own money, with their doctor's advice, to decide what care is best for them. This would increase competition among providers, lower prices, and offer patients more choice and involvement in their care.

2. Reform our tort laws. Doctors have a calling to help patients. But, as we all are human, we make mistakes. It is important that patients who are injured by medical mistakes be compensated as the law is supposed to allow. However, the law is supposed to be able to sort good healthcare from bad healthcare. Instead, it is run ad hoc, jury by jury, with no set standards. The system may favor a doctor even though a mistake was made, or it may favor a patient if no mistake was made. This unreliability leads to defensive medicine—doctors ordering tests and procedures just to prove that they did something, or excessively documenting trivial facts to prove they looked at everything. The cost of defensive medicine has been estimated up to $200 billion per year. The current laws neglect both the patient and the doctor and drive up costs with administrative and attorney fees.

Here is an example of defensive medicine. If a family physician determines a patient's headache is likely due to tension and there are no warning signs for something serious, the doctor may choose to not order a CT scan and have the patient follow up if symptoms do not improve. A tumor or bleeding in the brain could present in such a way despite a normal clinical evaluation by the doctor, but that's rare. If the patient does, in the end, have a tumor or bleeding, she can sue the doctor for not ordering the CT scan earlier. In turn, that doctor doesn't want that to ever happen again, even though he did everything right by using his clinical knowledge to determine nothing serious was likely going on. Thus, he will order CTs on everyone simply to avoid a lawsuit, even though he knows that the CT will be normal. This exponentially increases costs as doctors across the thousands of hospitals in America follow suit not only for headaches, but for other common ailments.

No, doctors cannot play God and know every outcome with the thousands of patients they see yearly. But they are good at using their knowledge and training to determine if someone is sick and likely needs further immediate attention.

Having said that, if the doctor did do something wrong, the patient is still taken advantage of with the current tort system. Thirty-nine percent of cases take three years to settle and 60 cents on the dollar are used for lawyer fees and administrative costs. Patients definitely deserve to be compensated for poor healthcare, and this current system fails them.

The answer rests in healthcare courts described by Common Good Chair Philip K. Howard. He states that expert judges without juries would determine what is good versus bad care. This would provide consistent standards of what is required in certain healthcare situations. It would benefit patients because they would not spend three years dealing with the jury system nor pay trial lawyers for a case they may not even win. And it would benefit physicians because they could act on their best professional judgment without being scared of being held liable when they did nothing wrong. It would let us do our jobs without being smothered by lawyers looking over our shoulder, yet provide patients with fair, consistent rulings in cases of being wronged.

By creating clear standards of care, healthcare courts will allow judges to dispose of weak and invalid claims quickly after filing, while also disincentivizing doctors and insurers from defending cases in which they are clearly at fault.

3. Increase patients' roles in their own health. This would lead to higher patient satisfaction and actually lower costs. This could be accomplished with health savings accounts. These accounts would be funded by patients with pre-tax dollars and contributions made by employers and/ or government subsidy stratified based on the individual's income and job status. With money in these accounts, patients would be able to discern costs better and use this money as if they were consuming any other good or service, such as handyman services. This money could grow each year like an investment account and even be passed on to heirs at the time of death, keeping that sense of ownership with loved ones.

For these accounts to work well, though, hospitals' and doctors' prices need to be more transparent and reflect true costs so patients know what they are buying. Currently, that is impossible. Hospital and doctor bills make little sense, are falsely inflated (as described earlier), and do not reflect true costs, leaving patients confused about real costs of their health.

When a patient hurts his knee and goes to the doctor, the doctor orders an expensive MRI with no mention of costs. The patient's insurance "covers" the MRI, making the costs a nonissue for that patient. There is no incentive to try ice, physical therapy, and rest before delving into an expensive MRI. If she knew the actual price for that MRI, the patient could know what she was "buying." This price would be significantly less than the inflated charges because prices would be required to be transparent. True prices would be published and patients could shop for MRI scanners just as they would for any other service. This would allow patients control over how they spend their healthcare dollars.

In the same light, during the last six months of our lives, we spend up to 50% of our own total lifetime healthcare dollars. In America, when patients are extremely sick and brought into the hospital, everything in our medical repertoire is used to keep them alive. Costs can be up to $10,000 per day of ICU care, not including other aggressive measures.

Unfortunately, patients may not know these costs. With patient-funded health savings accounts, patients would have more of a role in their own care and could decide based on a doctor's recommendation the best course of action, considering the patient's prognosis, benefits, risks, and costs. Of course, families always have input into their loved ones' health near the end of their life and can decide how aggressive they wish to be while talking with their team of doctors.

Doctors are not bringing up hospice to patients early enough. Instead, many families with their loved ones are faced spending their last months in an ICU, hooked up to breathing tubes, only prolonging the inevitable. Patients and their families are being deprived of spending that time at home in a more comfortable setting. Quality of life is not being brought up, only quantity. A February 17, 2012 article in *The Washington Post,* "An Unrealistic View of Death, Through a Doctor's Eyes," addresses these end-of-life issues extremely well.

The author states that modern medicine may be doing more to complicate end-of-life issues, rather than improve it. People think death is a failure of modern medicine rather than simply life's natural conclusion. I am not saying that every patient in an ICU needs to consider hospice. Each patient is unique and families should decide based on their values and wishes. A previously healthy 28-year-old involved in a car wreck who remains in an ICU may need months there to recover and would benefit from this long hospitalization. However, a 90-year-old patient with other medical problems such as heart failure and kidney disease in the ICU with a new diagnosis of a terminal cancer may benefit from a talk with hospice. Every human being is unique and families and doctors need to be more open about goals of care at the end of life

An interesting article by Ken Murray, MD, "How Doctors Die," details some of these issues (http://thehealthcareblog.com/blog/2012/08/06/how-doctors-die). Murray points out that most doctors choose less, not more, care at the end of their life because they personally witness the limits to human medicine. There is not always an answer or a cure and doing nothing is sometimes the best care available.

All in all, more patient ownership of end of life using their health savings accounts, combined with frank discussions with their doctors about these end-of-life issues, would lower healthcare costs and even help families cope with difficult illnesses. This explains why doctors choose a much less aggressive course near the end of their own lives—they know that some care is futile.

A December 17, 2013 article written by Dr. Jordan Grumet on KevinMD.com addresses this idea of futility of care, relating a mechanic to a doctor and healthcare.

Unlike Mechanics, Doctors Have Been Denied the Basic Logic of Futility

A guy has his car towed to the mechanic. All four tires are slashed. He has a simple request.

Please replace the tires.

But this is one of those comprehensive care mechanics. He not only examines the tires, he does a full once over. He pops the hood and immediately knows that the engine is shot. It's fried. The cost of fixing the engine is more than the value of the car. It's a zero sum game. The owner shouldn't replace the tires, he shouldn't work on the engine, and this car belongs in the scrap heap. He saunters out to the waiting room, and delivers the bad news to his eager customer. The mechanic is utterly stunned by what he hears next.

Please replace the tires.

The mechanic, being a kind and gentle sort, assumes that he has been misunderstood. He sits down quietly next to his fellow human being. He again explains, more slowly this time, how the cars value is minimal. He draws a diagram to demonstrate why the engine won't function. He reiterates the futility of changing the tires on such a car. It is not only a waste of money; it is a waste of precious time.

The customer turns his back to the mechanic, pulls out his mobile phone, and dials furtively. He hands the mechanic the phone. It's the customer's insurance agent.

Please replace the tires. We will cover it.

The office is full, the cars are piling up in the lot, and yet the mechanic patiently tries to explain the situation again. Again he tells how the engine is nonfunctional. Again he outlines the price of possible fixes and how they are completely cost prohibitive. The tires are just the icing on the cake. They are not the problem, and fixing them will solve nothing.

The customer snatches the mobile out of his hand and dials yet another number. He pushes the phone back without saying a word. This time it is a lawyer. He demands that the mechanic fix the tires unless he wants to face a lawsuit.

So the mechanic bills the insurance company. He replaces all four tires. He drops the car in the lot and gives the customer the keys. The customer thanks him, walks out to the car, gets in, and puts the keys in the ignition. Nothing happens. He gives it another try. Nothing happens. He walks back into the shop and approaches the mechanic with one more question.

How much will you charge me to tow this thing to the junk yard?

In reality, no mechanic would have been expected to fix the tires. No insurance company would have paid the bill. And no lawyer would have taken a case they so clearly couldn't win.

Yet doctors are expected to put dying patients on dialysis, give fourth line chemotherapy when the first three lines (which actually have some clinical benefit) fail, and refuse to turn off the battery of defibrillators in bed bound, obtunded, dementia patients.

We don't do this because we want to.

Unlike the mechanic, we have been denied the basic logic of futility.

Many patients' families want more and more done even though it is futile. However, with our culture in medicine of always appeasing the family members and patients, we deliver care that is likely futile on a daily basis. It costs hundreds of thousands of dollars and does nothing to prolong the patient's life. I believe that a lot of this type of care can be prevented if doctors had more frank discussions with their patients and their families about their prognosis. Now, this has nothing to do with "death panels" that were discussed in the media a few years ago. I'm not saying that really sick patients should be allowed to die. However, for those particular patients for whom doctors deem further care to be futile, frank discussions need to be initiated about prolonging life.

A few weekends ago when I was on call, I was paged for a constipation consult—one of about 15 consults that day. After delving into the chart and gathering the necessary information on this patient, I realized that this patient had stage four stomach cancer (metastatic) that spread to all parts of his body, including his abdomen. The cancer was actually wrapping around his bowels and kinking them off, preventing him from having a bowel movement. Surprisingly, in the preceding weeks, he was under the care of an oncologist, a cancer doctor who was administering chemotherapy.

I walked in the room and began to talk to the patient and his wife for the first time. After talking for about 10 minutes, I realized that this family was either in complete denial or did not know the stage of his cancer. The wife said, "I hope you can give him something for his constipation and fix it, so we can move on." I began to tell her my thoughts about how this cancer had spread based on the CT findings. Then, I realized she had no idea of the gravity of the situation. She believed he had a minor sickness with some constipation, when in reality, this gentleman had stage four cancer with a three-month prognosis. She replied, "No one ever mentioned the word 'spread' to me."

I ended up doing a colonoscopy on this patient, only to find a narrowing of his rectum due to the spread of this disease. In the end, we discussed hospice, but the fact that this family was unaware of the prognosis is alarming and represents a failure in our healthcare environment today. It shows that we as doctors need to make sure patients understand the gravity of their conditions early and give them options for their care, including hospice.

Dr. John Hunt, author of *Assume the Physician*, posted on KevinMD.com on December 21, 2013 an article about the concept of moral hazard. It exemplified this idea of why medical costs are increasing and are different than any other service in America:

> If you learn nothing else today, I would ask you to learn that *moral hazard* is the cause of medical price hyperinflation.
>
> Moral hazard is not just two words that don't seem to go together. Moral hazard is when the person who bears the economic burden of a decision is not the decision maker. In the health care setting, moral hazard is when the third party payer (insurance/government) bears the economic consequences of a patient's decision.
>
> When there is moral hazard, the patient cares less about what drugs or procedures cost, and cares less about what doctors charge. If the "buyer" does not sufficiently care what things cost, of course the prices rise. Why wouldn't they? If I could sell my 20-cent candy bar for $40 to the first person who comes in the door, why would I not charge $40? If everyone in America let their teenage daughters go shopping for clothes with ad lib unlimited access to the parent's credit card, think of the effects on the prices at stores such as the Gap and Abercrombie & Fitch. The prices would skyrocket.

High technology is not the cause of medical inflation: high tech in all private sectors of the economy, such as information technology, brings prices rapidly *down*, and it would do so in medicine but for moral hazard. Medical liability is a contributor to high costs, but again, if the patients bore the financial costs of the defensive medicine tests ordered by physicians, the patients would balk, and unnecessary defensive medicine would decline.

To address the price inflation caused by moral hazard, government mandates price controls, which always and absolutely lead to shortages and misallocation of resources and are uniformly and always proven to fail. We are in this stage currently in our country, with price controls dominating the medical landscape. And it is of course failing.

To reverse medical hyperinflation requires elimination of moral hazard. Either the patient has to pay for the care they choose, or insurance companies or the government that is paying will have to make the medical decisions for the patient. Both of these options eliminate moral hazard and both will bring down the prices of care. Nothing else will work. The important question therefore is not who should pay for health care, but rather who should be making your medical decisions? Do you want Obama making your personal medical decisions for you? Or should you make them yourself? If you think you should make your own medical decisions, then the only way to solve the economic failure of our medical system is for you to also pay your own medical bills.

Now, with health care prices so enormously overinflated, the concept of paying your own expenses is inconceivable. But again, if everyone pays for his own medical expenses, moral hazard goes away, and prices will fall every bit as fast and as far as the prices of computers has fallen. And think how accessible excellent computers are today. Low prices from the free market will make health care accessible and excellent and far more affordable. In contrast, health insurance makes health care impossibly expensive and it will decay into a situation in which the government will control personal medical decisions.

The cheapest form of health care is to let sick people die. And the government will always need to save money on health care so they can afford to send soldiers to foreign lands that have oil, subsidize big agribusiness to grow corn to make ethanol to destroy our engines, give huge grants to bankrupt companies whose executives support Obama, double the size of the NSA's Utah data center, or bail out a few more Wall Street looters.

Remember that health insurance—because of its inherent moral hazard—is the problem, not the solution.

Instead of letting the politicians tell us what to do, we should let the people figure it out in the marketplace of free ideas and free exchange. And as a critical part of this, those who care about the poor should be generous to the poor, directly and personally, as opposed to having their generosity channeled through the corruption of the crony-government coffers. Americans are as a whole the most generous people on the planet. And doctors are the most generous of Americans, or at least we used to be before we as a profession got so consumed and beaten down by the bureaucracy of health insurance and government. Don't let the government continue to abolish our culture of individual generosity.

We can solve our health care woes. The government can't. But we can.

4. Prevent chronic illnesses. Chronic illnesses such as heart disease and diabetes end up costing Americans a lot as they age. We are good at treating complex medical problems with patients who are very sick, but not very good at reducing medical costs through preventative medicine. We are good at bringing a new state of the art drug used to thin the blood to the market, but bad at actually preventing the reason for needing that drug in the first place!

In fact, 50% of our healthcare dollars ($623 billion) are spent on the sickest 5% of patients (30 million) in America, according to an article in the January 1, 2012 issue of USA TODAY (http://usatoday30.usatoday.com/news/washington/story/2012-01-11/health-care-costs-11/52505562/1). Interestingly, the top 1% of healthcare "spenders" accounted for 20% of the total healthcare expenditures in America. These are usually patients with multiple chronic medical conditions such as obesity, diabetes, kidney, and heart disease.

Studies often show that Americans spend a lot on healthcare, yet the United States is ranked lower than most other countries on healthcare outcomes. We spend a lot on patients who are very sick to prolong their life, but do little to prevent them from getting sick. When patients come from other countries to get treatment in the United States, this further exacerbates this concept by having to treat very sick patients who cannot be treated in other countries.

Sanjay Gupta summed up the solution to this paradox very well in a December 2, 2013 CNN article (www.cnn.com/2013/12/02/opinion/gupta-health-optimize). He states that increased access to healthcare with Obamacare would not improve our health outcomes. Rather, patients taking ownership of their own health and holding themselves accountable will promote a healthier America. Eating better, exercising more, and reducing stress can go a long way. It would also reduce the likelihood of developing these expensive chronic medical conditions, which drive costs higher.

A good example of preventing illness versus treating a costly illness at its end stage involves the new therapy for hepatitis C. This chronic disease causes 30% of patients to develop scarring (cirrhosis) of their liver over their lifetime. It is the number two reason for a costly liver transplant and patients often die from complications of the disease. Hepatitis C, if not treated, leads to other problems that cost our system tremendously, as these patients get cancer, bleed excessively which requires ICU care, and develop other conditions that land them in the hospital for days.

In 2014, many new drugs were FDA-approved for treating hepatitis C—a major breakthrough for a disease that kills so many. Unfortunately, despite these "miracle" drugs that could cure hepatitis C in two to three months, insurance companies balked at covering these medications. They thought the initial cost was too high despite the fact that it would save money long term and patients would not suffer the complications of the disease. That's just another example of us choosing the more expensive road in trying to treat a condition after it has wreaked havoc versus trying to prevent or cure it in the first place.

5. Reign in the number and salaries of hospital administrators. A May 17, 2014 *New York Times* article by Elisabeth Rosenthal summarizes this issue well (www.nytimes.com/2014/05/18/sunday-review/doctors-salaries-are-not-the-big-cost.html). Administrators have effectively shielded their large total compensation package (up to $36 million per year) and have used their negotiating power to pit the loss of health system revenue on doctors and their behaviors in care.

While reimbursement for office visits and procedures falls to less than 50% through many of the exchanges and other government-based programs such as Medicare and Medicaid, CEOs and hospital administrators continue to financially outpace their colleagues in other sectors of business. Yet, despite administrators' input and power, they never suffer from pay cuts due to low patient satisfaction scores. They never face lawsuits. They never wake up at 2:00 a.m. to save a patient's life. They never perform the life-saving procedures after being trained for 14 years. They don't even answer an email after 4:30 p.m. on a weeknight, let alone talk to a patient about their cancer diagnosis at 3:00 a.m. They suggest cutting healthcare staff such as nurses who get paid $26 per hour to save money, yet fail to mention that cutting one of their salaries of $263,000 (on average) would allow more nurses help those patients in need of care.

Doctors really do not even know what these administrators do all day. All we know is that they have offices twice the size and quality of ours, leave at 4:30 p.m. while we are still seeing patients, and get paid more than most doctors do, yet without the long work hours and training. Yet, ironically, the only reason the administrators have a job is because of doctors who take care of patients. The number of administrators has risen 2500% over the past decade while the number of doctors has risen by single-digit percentage points. In addition, these administrators command high salaries, leading to up to 30% of all healthcare costs. These administrators are simply contributing to the large overhead of a health system rather than cutting costs. When we simply need more doctors or support staff, they are creating more meaningless middle management jobs that do not directly affect patient care.

There are VPs of this and that. I am surprised there is not a Vice President of the East Wing restroom facility. If we work on reducing the number of these administrators and attempt to find those who have actually been involved in the front lines of care in the hospital, we will come a long way. This is hard to do, as these administrators are businesspeople skilled at lobbying, while doctors are too busy caring for the nation's sick. We need doctors to stand up for ourselves and our patients and get Washington to hear our voices as well.

Final Words

In conclusion, I believe that Capitol Hill needs input from doctors working on the front lines to discuss our issues so that the best reform possible can be made. Doctors experience all of the above issues on a daily basis and have insight that politicians cannot have.

I believe that by empowering patients more in the healthcare system through health savings accounts, reforming our tort laws, making costs more transparent, being more realistic about end-of-life issues, and living healthier, we can create a system that can benefit everyone.

I hope this book, as a personal account of the past 15 years of my life as a doctor in training, is useful and used for many purposes.

I hope that it inspires young bright minds to pursue medicine, as being a doctor is the greatest privilege in the world.

I hope that it helps the public and future leaders realize the long journey we endure so health policy changes can be made with input from doctors themselves.

I hope it inspires and educates patients so they know we make sacrifices every day and put our heart, mind, and soul into making them healthier.

And finally, I hope that it redirects criticisms and perceptions of doctors from being well-oiled, omnipotent, emotionless, debt-free machines, into normal people who worked hard in life, have families, and have the same emotions and weaknesses as everyone else.

We are expected to work 30-hour shifts and work well over 80 hours per week, not sleep every fourth night in training, be compassionate toward patients even if they are frustrated, answer their phone calls at all hours of the day, risk lawsuits, take on mountains of debt, and lose out on our 20s to textbooks and hospitals, all for the privilege of making our patients' lives healthier.

We are forced to listen to the media saying that we make too much money even though they have never lived a day in the life of a doctor. They do not have our debt load. They do not have our responsibility of a patient's life in their hands daily. They do not get bodily fluids/matter all over them daily. They don't have to deliver bad news to patients daily or deal with sick and vulnerable patients. They do not have to call patients at night or on their ride home from work. They do not have to risk lawsuits if things go poorly despite their best intentions. They do not wake up to a pager at all hours of the night and then work the next day. No, all they can do is google our salaries and say we make a lot of money without putting it into context.

In addition to the media, we must listen to hospital administrators tell us to see more patients per hour, yet get paid less and less. They tell us to improve our patient satisfaction scores, even though no study shows that better scores mean better care. They tell us that their health system is losing money, yet their bonuses and offices get bigger. We hear them call us "healthcare providers," not doctors. They reduce us to a number, a person who can be easily replaced, a cog in the wheel, a robot. While we physicians are crammed into rooms that barely fit four physicians, we watch our administrators enjoy their own spacious offices. They do not know the sanctity of saving a life or answering calls at all hours of the day. They work 8:00 a.m. to 4:30 p.m. They dress in nice suits, not scrubs that are spattered with blood and saliva from a patient. And they do not take call.

We as doctors care for our patients because we have a calling—a calling that we hope we can uphold despite the constant onslaught from administrators, insurance companies, and the media trying to control us and demonize us.

I leave you with a KevinMD.com entry from August 21, 2011 from a patient, Rachel Loa, who wrote in response to an article on how doctors need to save the costs of Medicare. It is fitting that I end with an anecdote from a patient because in the end, this is the reason we went into medicine: to care for our patients with our mind, heart, and soul.

> As a patient, and reader of KevinMD.com, I'd like to respond to a recent piece, "Doctors face difficult choices to save Medicare."
>
> The funny thing about this entire situation is that people refer to numbers. Numbers that consist of how much doctors are in debt when actually entering into the working world, how much Medicare reimburses or pays annually, how many patients are actually on Medicare, and how much in debt our country truly is. The bottom line is that these physicians are the soul of our country.

These [doctors] are the men and women in this country that spend years in school learning how to save lives and take care of some of the most unruly and agonizing patients in the world. Our country fails to view these physicians as people as well. We expect these men and women to work around the clock to take care of us, individually, with patience, understanding, and knowledge. Expertise in their field that is questioned every day—questioned and denied by insurance companies that believe that they have a say in what medication is necessary for patients. Insurance companies that have now been given the power to make decisions for patients with absolutely no medical knowledge or background, but simply based off of a number step-edit system.

These doctors, these physicians, these people, have families that they rarely see. Have lives that they are barely able to live because despite what our country may believe, these men and women have now been forced to work around the clock simply to make a living that merely pays off what they initially set out to do. These people essentially give their lives away to the number of patients demanding instant results and instantaneous fixes to health problems related to their own decisions and the ways in which they have chosen to live. Regardless of the quality of patients in our country, or our lack to initiate any sort of self-help, these men and women still believe it is their responsibility to provide, provide, provide, as we continue to demand, demand, demand.

In no way do we apply, give thanks, or attribute the respect that these physicians deserve to them regularly. Instead we threaten their practices, their homes, their integrity and we question their desire to practice medicine; which is perhaps one of the most dangerous things that we as a country can do.

When we demoralize these physicians, we show no respect for their hard work, for their lives being given up to take care of sometimes fifty to sixty strangers a day, then we give up on the survival of humanity. We give up on the people that provide regularly and we give up on the best healthcare system in the world. With lowering our respect for physicians, and only increasing our uncontrolled, invaluable ability to self-proclaim what we as individuals believe that we deserve, we put these men and women in extremely compromising positions. Positions that not only will cause them despise their patience, despise healthcare, but to ultimately despise the practice of medicine; if we continue down this path, our physicians will no longer be practicing for the right reasons, our doctors will no longer desire to have educations that place them hundreds of thousands of dollars in debt, and we will no longer uphold the strongest medicinal system in the world. We will fall, and we will suffer and we will hurt, because there will not be anyone on the other side to take care of us once it is all said and done.